your guide to

coeliac disease

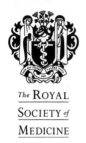

The ROYAL
SOCIETY of
MEDICINE

your guide to

coeliac
disease

Professor Peter Howdle
BSc, MD, FRCP

Hodder Arnold

A MEMBER OF THE HODDER HEADLINE GROUP

Hodder Arnold have agreed to pay 50 pence per product on all sales made of this title to the retailer at a discount of up to and including 60% from the UK Recommended Retail Price to Coeliac UK.

Orders: Please contact Bookpoint Ltd, 130 Milton Park, Abingdon, Oxon OX14 4SB. Telephone: (44) 01235 827720, Fax: (44) 01235 400454. Lines are open from 9.00 to 18.00, Monday to Saturday, with a 24-hour message answering service. You can also order through our website www.hoddereducation.com

British Library Cataloguing in Publication Data
A catalogue record for this title is available from the British Library.

ISBN-10: 0 340 928859
ISBN-13: 9 780340 928851

First published	2007			
Impression number	10 9 8 7 6 5 4 3 2 1			
Year	2010	2009	2008	2007

Typeset by Servis Filmsetting Limited, Longsight, Manchester. Printed in Great Britain for Hodder Arnold, a division of Hodder Headline, 338 Euston Road, London NW1 3BH, by Cox & Wyman Ltd, Reading, Berkshire.

Hodder Headline's policy is to use papers that are natural, renewable and recyclable products and made from wood grown in sustainable forests. The logging and manufacturing processes are expected to conform to the environmental regulations of the country of origin.

Every effort has been made to trace copyright for material used in this book. The authors and publishers would be happy to make arrangements with any holder of copyright whom it has not been possible to trace successfully by the time of going to press.

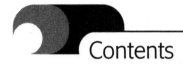
Contents

Acknowledgements

To Susan, for her unfailing support and love over many years.

Particular thanks are due to Coeliac UK for allowing me to use much of their advice for patients and carers.

Especial thanks are due to Mrs Eileen Tasker, not only for all her secretarial help, but also for her support and friendship over many years.

The author and publishers would also like to thank the following organizations for permission to reproduce material in this book:

Elsevier Ltd for Plates 3, 4, 6 and 7 (reprinted from *Encyclopedia of Food Sciences* and *Nutrition* (2nd edition) by Caballero, Trugo and Finglass (eds), 2003, p. 990) and Plates 11 and 12 (reprinted from *Malabsorption in Clinical Practice* by Losowsky, Kelleher and Walker, 1974, p. 193); Blackwell Scientific Publications for Figures 3.4, 5.2 and Plate 10 (reprinted from *Coeliac Disease* by Marsh (ed.), 1992, pp. 306, 155 and 52 respectively); and Coeliac UK for Plate 10.

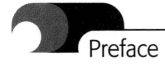 Preface

This new book, published in partnership with the Royal Society of Medicine, provides detailed, useful and up-to-date information on coeliac disease. It contains expert yet user-friendly advice, with such useful features as:

Key Terms: demystifying the jargon
Questions and Answers: answering the burning questions
Myths and Facts: debunking the misconceptions
My Experience: how it feels to live with, or care for someone with, this condition.

Bearing the hallmark of excellence and accessibility that characterizes the work of the Royal Society of Medicine, this important guide will enable you and your family to gain some control over the way your coeliac disease is managed by being better informed.

Peter Richardson
Director of Publications
Royal Society of Medicine

Introduction

I was pleased to be asked by the Royal Society of Medicine and the publishers to write this book since I have been looking after coeliac patients for almost 30 years and, during that time, have got to know many of them very well and have learnt so much from them. I have also spent a lot of time researching into various aspects of coeliac disease and discussing results of research with many colleagues around the world. I have been a medical adviser to Coeliac UK for many years, and am grateful to the staff there for helpful advice during the writing of this book. Coeliac UK started as a small self-help group for coeliac patients more than 35 years ago and has now grown into a strong and important organization to support people with coeliac disease and dermatitis herpetiformis. It is one of the best national societies in the world for patients with coeliac disease.

This book is for patients and their carers, family and friends who want to know more about coeliac disease. I hope it will make some things clearer and give the reader greater understanding and reassurance. Professional colleagues may also find it helpful when they are advising patients and their carers.

The book begins with a brief introduction and history of coeliac disease. There then follows a description – as simple as I can make it – of the background science about how the bowel is made and works. There are chapters describing how the disease shows itself and how it is diagnosed and, finally, what to do about it, particularly concerning the special diet. If there are words you do not fully understand, please refer to the glossary at the end of the book.

How people cope with all this depends upon themselves, their carers, family and friends. I have tried to be positive and reassuring, since so many of my patients lead very fulfilling and busy lives, despite having coeliac disease. One lady was diagnosed when she was in her early eighties. She took to the diet very well and she and her husband still went walking on Ilkley Moor – the only thing she gave up was potholing!

Professor Peter Howdle
Professor of Clinical Medicine
Consultant Gastroenterologist
St. James's University Hospital
Leeds

CHAPTER

1

What is coeliac disease?

Introduction

Coeliac disease is a fascinating disease to describe and to understand. As you will see from reading this book, it is a medical condition in which the bowel is affected as a result of exposure to a common ingredient of the normal diet. Our understanding of how this happens has increased in recent years, but why it occurs is still largely an enigma. We certainly know that **wheat** and related products are involved, and that the condition is much more common than previously realized. In people who are affected there is a variety of symptoms, many of which are from the **gastrointestinal tract**.

The scientific study of the disease has led to a much deeper understanding of how the immune system of the intestine works. Despite the many unanswered questions, it is one of the few diseases which can be treated satisfactorily by

wheat
A plant of the grass family. It is cultivated for its seeds which, when milled, constitute flour. A good source of nutrition, particularly carbohydrate, for humans.

gastrointestinal tract
The long, flexible muscular tube which goes from the mouth to the anus. It includes the gullet, the stomach and the bowel (intestine). It allows food and drink to be digested and absorbed, and the waste to be passed out of the body.

dietary means and, fortunately, almost all diagnosed and treated patients lead normal lives provided they keep to the diet.

The history of coeliac disease

Coeliac is an unusual word (pronounced 'see-lee-ack'), and derives from a Greek word meaning 'belonging to the belly' or 'suffering in the bowels'. It is claimed to have first been used for a medical condition by Aretaeus from Cappadocia (now part of modern Turkey) who worked as a doctor in Rome in the second century AD. He described an illness with recurrent diarrhoea, wind and a rumbling abdomen (belly), so he could well have been describing patients with coeliac disease! In those days little was known about the disease or its treatment, but Aretaeus did say 'The illness is protracted and difficult to cure for even if it seems to have ceased it recurs without apparent cause and even a slight dietary error can lead to relapse.'

However, it was not until 1888 that the first accurate description of coeliac disease was published by Dr Samuel Gee. He was a consultant at St Bartholomew's Hospital in London and he wrote a short medical paper which is remarkably accurate, even today when we know so much more about coeliac disease. Samuel Gee's name will probably be known to some older readers, as there used to be a patent cough medicine called 'Gee's Linctus'.

Gee had obviously observed his patients very carefully, since his description cannot be bettered. He wrote of 'a kind of chronic indigestion' affecting people of all ages, with diarrhoea, weight loss, wasting of the muscles and weakness as part of a relapsing illness. He did not know the cause, but said that 'if the patient can be cured at all, it must be by means of diet.' Gee even described treating a child with best Dutch mussels each day, who improved enormously, but relapsed when the season for mussels was over!

Over the next 60 years other doctors diagnosed the disease without knowing the cause. Several tried altering the diet, and sometimes this worked. For example, there was the famous 'banana diet' used in children successfully prior to and during the Second World War. I remember my mother recounting how children with the condition were given special banana rations during the war and public appeals for bananas were made. Nowadays we can understand how these diets helped, since they were providing different sources of nourishment which largely avoided bread.

In 1950 Willem Dicke, a children's specialist in Holland, showed that the condition of children who had symptoms of coeliac disease improved by removing wheat from their diet. Dicke and his fellow workers went on to show that it was a part of the wheat called **gluten** which was responsible for provoking the symptoms in their coeliac patients. The story is told that Dicke suggested wheat was involved, since during the Second World War he had noticed that coeliac children improved when wheat and rye were unavailable in Holland but that after the war, when these crops were once again available, the children relapsed.

Two other major advances were made in our understanding of coeliac disease during the 1950s. Dr John Paulley, a physician in Ipswich, showed in 1954 that the lining of the upper part

gluten
The protein in the wheat seed which provides amino acids for the growing plant, or for a human being when used as food. It provides much of the texture of flour when cooked.

of the bowel was abnormal in coeliac patients. He did this by obtaining pieces of the intestine from coeliac patients when they were undergoing abdominal operations since, in those days, there was no other way of obtaining a fresh piece (**biopsy**) of the intestine to examine under a microscope.

biopsy
A small piece of tissue taken for laboratory examination to help with diagnosis or assessment of treatment.

However, in 1956 in London, Dr Margot Shiner developed a biopsy tube which could be passed through the mouth and down into the stomach and beyond. Although very crude by modern standards, this did allow biopsies to be obtained from the intestine. Soon afterwards, in 1957 in America, Dr Crosby developed the 'Crosby capsule'. Many older patients will remember this. It was like a large lozenge on the end of a thin plastic tube. The lozenge was swallowed and allowed to pass out of the stomach and into the intestine. Its position was checked by an X-ray and then suction was applied on the plastic tube at the mouth. This suction fired a blade in the capsule, which caught a biopsy. The capsule was then pulled out. As you can imagine, it was not a very pleasant experience, especially since the whole procedure could take some hours.

These three important advances in the 1950s make this a significant decade for the study of coeliac disease.

To summarize: wheat was found to be the ingredient causing coeliac disease, the main abnormality in the body being produced by the wheat was shown to be in the lining of the upper intestine, and a way of obtaining samples of the lining, without operation, for analysis was devised.

Later in this book many more advances will be described, and we now know more about which people may develop coeliac disease from a

genetic point of view. We know more about which part of wheat and related **cereals** causes the disease, and how that happens. We can also obtain biopsies much more easily with modern **endoscopes** and can assess the range of abnormalities seen in these biopsies from coeliac patients.

Knowing about many of these factors allows us to define coeliac disease more accurately. So, what is a modern definition of coeliac disease?

Coeliac disease is a permanent condition, principally affecting the small intestine in genetically predisposed individuals, which is precipitated by the ingestion of the gluten fraction of wheat and of the closely related cereals, *rye* and *barley*.

This leads us to various questions about the symptoms, the effects on the body, and the diet. Many of these questions will be answered in the following chapters of this book.

Terms used to denote coeliac disease

Arising out of the history of coeliac disease, and also the definition which has emerged, many names or terms have been used for the condition. Some of these are listed below:

◆ coeliac disease
◆ celiac disease (American spelling)
◆ coeliac sprue (sprue is a Dutch word meaning ulcers or inflammation)
◆ celiac sprue
◆ coeliac condition
◆ idiopathic sprue

genetics
The study of how we inherit characteristics from one generation to the next, through our genes.

cereal
A plant of the grass family which has been developed through evolution and plant breeding to produce seeds which are used as foods.

endoscope
A flexible fibre-optic instrument used to examine the inside of the gastrointestinal tract. It is passed through the mouth in order to see the oesophagus (gullet), stomach and duodenum (upper part of the small intestine). A moving television picture of the inside of these organs is seen.

rye
A similar plant to wheat; its seeds are also grown to produce food.

barley
A similar plant to wheat; its seeds are grown for food and also for the production of alcoholic drinks (beers, lagers).

✧ non-tropical sprue

✧ gluten sensitivity (referring to the part of wheat which provokes the condition)

✧ gluten sensitive enteropathy (referring to the damage to the bowel)

✧ gluten intolerance

✧ idiopathic steatorrhea (referring to the symptom of fatty diarrhoea)

✧ malabsorption syndrome (referring to the poor absorption of food constituents)

✧ Gee's disease (referring to Samuel Gee)

In the United Kingdom the name coeliac disease is most frequently used. The word 'coeliac' has become embedded in our medical terminology and is part of our medical tradition. As a means of communicating about the disease, it is clearly understood. Some treated patients are so well that they consider themselves as normal, and so prefer to call it the coeliac 'condition' rather than disease, which implies a chronic illness. However, coeliac disease is the term we most commonly use in the United Kingdom. An understandable reason for this is that the term 'disease' alerts doctors and patients to the possibility of complications, especially if there are dietary lapses.

gluten-sensitive enteropathy
An alternative name for coeliac disease, often used in North America.

In the United States, '**gluten-sensitive enteropathy**' (GSE) is frequently used. As can be seen from the definition of the disease, this term seeks to convey quite accurately its basis, in that it describes gluten causing a disease of the intestine (an 'enteropathy'). Americans often use less traditional terms and it is not surprising that GSE has found wide acceptance and usage. In this book, however, the term coeliac disease is used.

CHAPTER

2

The normal gut and the coeliac gut – what is abnormal?

The gastrointestinal tract

Coeliac disease is a disease in which the principal effects are seen in the intestine, even though, as will become evident from the following chapters, many parts of the body can be affected. It is important, therefore, to understand the structure of the gut, i.e. the gastrointestinal tract, and how it works. It is complicated!

In simple terms the gut starts at the mouth and continues, as the **oesophagus** or gullet, into the stomach (see Figure 2.1). From there it continues as the small intestine, a concertina-like tube divided into three continuous parts, called the **duodenum**, the **jejunum** and the **ileum**. The small intestine is estimated to be approximately 6 metres long on average in adults. The duodenum is usually about 20 centimetres in length, but the jejunum and ileum are much longer, at 2.4 metres and 3.6 metres respectively. These three

oesophagus (the gullet)
The first part of the gastrointestinal tract from the mouth to the stomach.

duodenum
The first part of the small intestine, just past the stomach.

jejunum
The mid-part of the small intestine, between the duodenum and the ileum.

ileum
The last part of the small intestine which joins on to the large intestine (or colon).

colon
The last part of the intestinal tract, also called the large intestine. It is about 1.5 metres long and joins the small intestine to the anus.

myth
The small intestine is small.

fact
The small intestine is very long (about 6 metres in adults) but it is a narrower tube than the 'large' intestine (or colon) so that is why it is called 'small'. Incidentally, the large intestine is much shorter (at 1.5 metres) than the small intestine.

small intestine
The long, flexible, muscular tube, about 6 metres long, which lies coiled up in the abdomen joining the stomach to the colon; its main function is to allow food to be digested and absorbed into the body.

mucosa
The innermost layer of the intestine, consisting of fine blood vessels, fine nerves, immune cells and connecting tissue; covered by the epithelium.

parts are very similar in structure. One follows the other and together they form a long continuous flexible tube which eventually joins the large (i.e. wider) intestine, or **colon**. This is a similar flexible tubular structure, which is much shorter (1.5 metres), but wider than the small intestine. Its final part is called the rectum, which finishes with the anal canal. It is in the small intestine where the typical abnormality of coeliac disease is seen.

Q **How does all the intestine fit into my body?**

A Your intestine (including the small intestine and the large intestine, or colon) is approximately 8 metres long. It is very soft and flexible and easily bends and folds. When you were a foetus and then a baby it grew and developed, and folded itself so that it fits snugly inside the abdomen. At certain points along its length it is fixed to the walls of the abdomen by body tissues, so that it cannot uncoil or twist in funny ways.

The structure of the small intestine

The **small intestine** is a long, flexible tube normally curled up within the abdomen (see Figure 2.1). Its wall is made up of four layers (see Figure 2.2): an outer or covering coat, called the serosa, beneath which there is a muscular layer; the third layer consists of a variety of cells and tissues called the submucosa, which supports the innermost layer which lines the lumen (the hollow centre) of the intestine and is called the **mucosa**. The mucosa contains many specialized cells and structures, including the

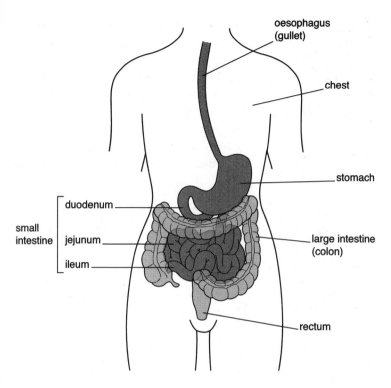

oesophagus
(gullet)

chest

stomach

duodenum

small
intestine

jejunum

large intestine
(colon)

ileum

rectum

▌ Figure 2.1 The gastrointestinal tract within the body.

epithelium which is the layer of cells lining its surface. These absorb and secrete products essential to maintain life. In the small intestine the mucosa is formed into finger-shaped projections called **villi**, which dramatically increase its surface area.

It is possible to see into the lumen (the interior) using an endoscope (see Plate 1). One can see that the muscle coat forms obvious rings around the intestine, but at this magnification it is not easy to see the villi. However, a small piece

epithelium
The layer of cells which covers the inside surface of the intestine.

villus (plural villi)
A finger-like projection of the small intestinal mucosa.

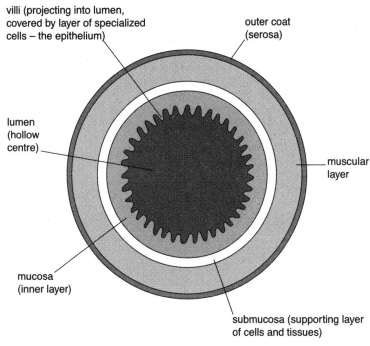

villi (projecting into lumen,
covered by layer of specialized
cells – the epithelium)

outer coat
(serosa)

lumen
(hollow
centre)

muscular
layer

mucosa
(inner layer)

submucosa (supporting layer
of cells and tissues)

❚ Figure 2.2 The layers of the wall of the small intestine.

(2–3mm) of the mucosa (a biopsy) can easily be taken (see Plate 2) and, under a magnifying glass, it is possible to see the villi as finger- or leaf-shaped projections (see Plate 3).

my experience

When I was first diagnosed with coeliac disease I saw a specialist at the clinic and also a dietitian. I came away with my head spinning. I could not take it all in and was almost frightened to eat. Fortunately the dietitian had given me some specimen diet sheets, so I stuck to those until I got more information about gluten-free foods.

My GP was most helpful in explaining how my body works; I never thought about it before. Apparently, the food we eat goes down into the stomach. In the stomach it is liquidized and then goes through the outlet of the stomach into the intestine. This has many fancy names, but is really a long, flexible, muscular tube, like the extendable pipe on a vacuum cleaner! The intestine is about nine metres long and is coiled up inside the tummy. It eventually ends in the bottom, at the anus, and that is where the waste comes out.

What surprised me is that all our food is broken down in the intestine into very small particles. These are then able to go from the intestine into the rest of the body. These small particles are reconstituted, mainly by the liver, to keep replenishing our bodily organs and provide us with energy.

Those of us with coeliac disease react to one of the parts of wheat, called gluten. This reaction damages the lining on the inside surface of the intestine. It then becomes inflamed and does not work properly, so we can get diarrhoea as the food is rushed through and not broken down properly. We can also lose weight and become anaemic because our food does not get from the intestine to the rest of the body. Naturally, if we don't eat wheat, the body can't react against it and eventually it returns to normal. We can then use all other foods normally, and remain well.

It's simple, isn't it? However, I asked my doctor why people get it – that's not so simple. Apparently it's partly to do with our genes (isn't everything these days?), but that is not the whole answer. I expect one day someone will find the answer.

Histological (under the microscope) examination of the small intestine

When a biopsy of the lining of the bowel has been taken, it is cut into thin, vertical sections, mounted on a glass slide and stained with various dyes to show up under a microscope. The report of what is seen is called a **histological** report. Plate 4 shows a photograph of normal mucosa seen

histology
The study under the microscope of thin slivers of biological samples, including biopsies of human tissue.

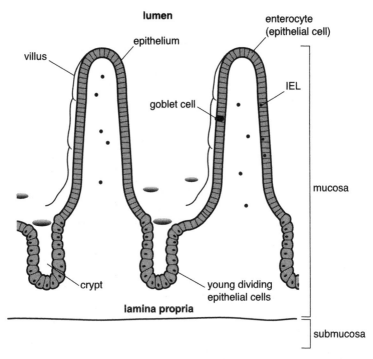

Figure 2.3 The normal mucosa showing the villi and crypts covered by the epithelium.

down a microscope. The finger-shaped villi can clearly be seen, covered by the epithelium – the layer of specialized cells particularly involved in absorbing nutrients. Figure 2.3 shows a diagram of the mucosa showing the structure of the villi. Villi are between 0.5 mm and 1 mm in height.

As can be seen from the diagram, the mucosa consists of the epithelium, i.e. the surface layer of cells, and the underlying tissue, called the '**lamina propria**'. This contains supporting fibres, fine nerves, blood vessels, lymph vessels and numerous cells mainly concerned with the immune system. This lamina propria is very active, keeping the mucosa healthy. Between the

lamina propria
The tissue of the mucosa which forms the core of the villi and surrounds the crypts.

villi are crevices called **crypts**. These are the places where the epithelial cells develop and mature. Crypt cells divide quite rapidly all the time to produce new epithelial cells, which are always moving up the crypt wall and onto the villous surface. When they reach the tip of the villus, they are sloughed off. This whole process, from production to death of the epithelial cells, takes between three and five days. Hence the epithelium is always renewing itself. Because the intestine is a three-dimensional structure, each villus will be surrounded around its base by several crypts, and those crypts will be supplying epithelial cells to several surrounding villi.

The main function of the epithelial cells, called **enterocytes**, is to absorb nutrients. Scattered amongst the enterocytes are goblet cells which produce mucus – a protective material for the surface of the epithelium. Also scattered between enterocytes are some immune cells called **lymphocytes**, the so-called IELs or 'intra-epithelial lymphocytes'.

The enterocyte is a rectangular cell and is joined quite tightly to its neighbours. It is interesting that the surface of each enterocyte, where absorption takes place, is itself made up of fine projections called 'microvilli', which can only be seen using an electron microscope (Plate 5). Because of all the folds, villous projections and microvilli, the overall surface area of the small intestine is as large as a tennis court!

How does the whole intestine work?

The mouth is important in preparing food for **digestion**. Chewing and mixing food with

crypt
A crevice in the mucosa between villi, where the epithelium develops.

enterocyte
A cell of the small intestinal epithelium which specializes in absorbing food constituents.

lymphocyte
A cell of the immune system which reacts against foreign substances in order to protect the body; there are several different types of lymphocyte.

intra-epithelial lymphocyte (IEL)
A lymphocyte within the small intestinal epithelium, between the enterocytes.

digestion
The liquidization and breakdown, within the lumen (i.e. the hollow centre) of the intestine, of food into smaller parts by specific chemicals (enzymes) produced by the body. This enables it to be absorbed into the body for nutrition and energy.

Q How long does food take to go through the intestine?

A This can vary from several hours to several days. However, studies show that if 20 small plastic beads are swallowed and followed through the intestine by taking X-rays, on average it takes three to four days for all of them to pass right through, although half will have passed in two days.

peristalsis
The normal forward movement of propulsion by the intestine, produced by its muscle layer.

saliva allows it to pass easily, on swallowing, down the oesophagus and into the stomach. The stomach is like a hopper, where food is mixed and liquidized with acid and enzymes. It is released in a regulated fashion out of the stomach into the small intestine. Here it is further digested and absorbed into the body for nutrition. Indigestible food constituents are passed through the small intestine into the colon, still in a liquidized form. In the colon, water is absorbed and solid waste matter is produced, which is passed when the bowels are opened. It is evident that once swallowing has started the contents of the intestinal tract need to move down. This happens by a process called '**peristalsis**' – the continuous involuntary muscular activity of the muscle layers of the intestine which keep the contents moving downwards through the whole length of the gut.

Q Can we live without our intestine?

A We can live without a large intestine (colon) as many people do who have had the colon removed for colitis. In these patients, the small intestine is then reconnected to the anus, if possible, but usually ends instead in a 'stoma', an opening through the abdominal wall onto the skin, and empties into a specially designed bag. If some of the small intestine has to be removed or is severely diseased, enough healthy small intestine has to remain to allow absorption of adequate nutrition from the diet; the minimum length required is about one metre. If there is less than this, the patient would require permanent feeding into a vein. This is possible but is very complicated. So, we cannot live completely without an intestine unless we can obtain nutrition into a vein.

myth
Our intestines are normally free of infection.

fact
That is true in the sense that normally we do not have gastroenteritis caused by bugs. However, much of the lining of the intestine, especially of the large intestine, is home for millions of harmless bugs, with which we live in harmony. These are in fact important to keep things working normally.

What does the small intestine do?

As we have just seen, one of its functions is to play its part in propelling its contents downwards: peristalsis. Two other very important functions are the digestion and **absorption** of food.

Food consists mainly of fats, proteins, carbohydrates, vitamins, minerals and indigestible fibre. The structure of the small intestine and related organs is designed for these processes of digestion and absorption. As seen in Figure 2.4, the first part of the small intestine is the duodenum, which is high inside the abdomen, just under the right ribs, and curves around the pancreas. The pancreas empties the digestive juices (enzymes) it produces into the duodenum, so that these enzymes can break down the food.

The duct from the pancreas is joined by the bile duct from the gall bladder and liver. The bile contains bile acids (sometimes called bile salts). These act as a detergent to dissolve the fat (just like washing-up liquid dissolves fat when washing-up). Once dissolved in this way, the fatty breakdown products are absorbed across the surface of the enterocytes (the epithelial cells) and pass through these cells into the blood

absorption
The transfer of food constituents from the lumen (i.e. the hollow centre) of the small intestine, across the epithelium and into the body, for use as nutrition and energy.

Q **How quickly do we absorb our food?**

A Once we have swallowed our food it is liquidized in the stomach and gradually released into the small intestine where it is broken down, and absorption into the body begins. All this starts as soon as we have eaten, but of course digestion and absorption depend upon the type of food and the amount. However, within minutes absorption will have started even though it may take several hours to complete.

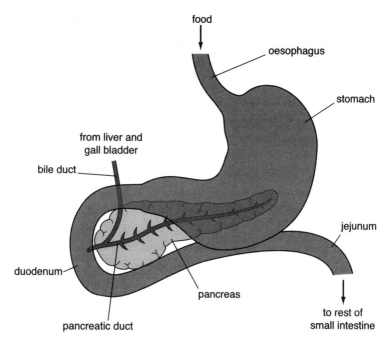

food

oesophagus

stomach

from liver and
gall bladder

bile duct

jejunum

duodenum

pancreas

to rest of
small intestine

pancreatic duct

Figure 2.4 The relationship of the duodenum and associated organs.

vessels and lymph vessels, where they are taken to the liver to be used for energy.

The enterocyte surface is also involved in the final digestion as well as the absorption of carbohydrates and proteins. The microvilli contain enzymes which break down the sugars and proteins into their smallest molecules. These are absorbed into the enterocytes and then passed via the blood vessels from the mucosa up to the liver, also to be used for energy or stored.

Although these digestive and absorptive processes begin in the duodenum with the addition of pancreatic enzymes and bile acids, they continue right throughout the small intestine. Hence its large surface area is very important for adequate nutrition. The other food constituents, such as minerals and vitamins, do not require breaking down but are absorbed by a variety of specific mechanisms across the enterocyte surfaces.

> **myth**
> Indigestion means we do not obtain any goodness from our food.

> **fact**
> Indigestion is a word many people use for describing a variety of symptoms related to eating food. Sometimes it means pain, or sickness, or wind, or bloating. It very rarely means that the intestine is unable to digest and absorb food adequately. It can, however, reflect a medical problem such as a stomach ulcer, or inflammation of the stomach.

> **myth**
> People are overweight because they absorb their food better.

> **fact**
> There is no evidence of this. Everyone varies in how much food they need for the energy they use. Unfortunately, overweight people eat more food than they actually need, and the excess is stored by the body for future use if required.

The other functions of the small intestine are *secretory* and *immunological*. The epithelium secretes mucus which acts as a protective barrier particularly against infections.

The gut is part of the **immune system** of the body and is, in fact, very sophisticated in this regard. In human beings the immune system is very complicated, but essentially its purpose is to protect us against 'foreign' substances, i.e. substances which are not part of ourselves. The immune system recognizes these foreigners and tries to eliminate them so, for example, if bacteria (bugs) get into our bodies, chemicals and cells are produced which engulf the bugs and kill them.

> **immune system**
> The body's mechanism for protecting itself against 'foreign' substances.

There is an important exception, however, since all the food that we eat is foreign and we do not reject it, usually! The immune system in the gut has developed so that it does not, in general, react against most foods. This is called 'oral tolerance'. Obviously some people do develop a specific immune reaction against certain substances, for example, nut allergy. Other food intolerances may be immunological, but often they are not.

The gut immune system

The immune system in the gut is very similar throughout, but here we are concentrating on the small intestine. We have already seen (Figure 2.3) that the mucosa has a villous structure, comprising of a lamina propria covered by an epithelial layer.

Innate immunity

The first immune defence is the layer of mucus on the surface of the epithelial cells. This contains some specific immunoglobulins (see below) but only provides limited protection.

The epithelial cells themselves and also other cells in the lamina propria beneath produce a variety of chemicals which are anti-bacterial. These defences are called 'innate immunity'.

Acquired immunity

antigen
A foreign substance, mainly protein, against which an antibody is specifically made by one's own body. Very occasionally the substance against which the antibody is made is not 'foreign' but part of the body itself (this is then an auto-antigen).

Apart from these innate defences, the immune system is able to learn to react very specifically against a particular foreign substance (an **'antigen'**) and always remembers to recognize this. This is called 'acquired immunity'. However, it is very complicated.

The acquired immune reaction begins when a foreign substance (antigen) is engulfed by a special cell which breaks it up and puts a part of it on its own surface. This is called antigen-presentation. It allows the lymphocytes to recognize the antigen as foreign and therefore to begin to react against it. This reaction involves the lymphocytes in multiplying and secreting chemicals to get rid of the antigen. One group of chemicals which is produced is the **immunoglobulins**. These recognize the antigen and help to eliminate it and, because they act specifically against the antigen, they are called '**antibodies**'. The immunoglobulins are of three main types: immunoglobulins A, G or M (IgA, IgG, IgM).

When the acquired immune system is acting in the gut, the process we have just described takes place in the mucosa. The immunoglobulin produced by the lymphocytes in the gut is IgA.

As mentioned above, fortunately the gut immune system does not normally mount immune reactions against food substances, even though these are foreign. The reasons for this oral tolerance are complex, but depend upon early exposure to particular food, and the amount taken. The immune system learns to suppress the lymphocytes. Occasionally, however, certain foods are not tolerated and a reaction with clinical symptoms occurs.

The other important feature to remember about the immune system is that it is aimed at foreign material and hence it does not attack the body's own tissues. In some diseases, however, this does happen. These are called **autoimmune diseases** (an example is rheumatoid arthritis, where the lymphocytes attack the lining of the joints).

The coeliac gut

Although there has been a long explanation of the normal structure and function of the gut,

immunoglobulin
A chemical produced by a type of lymphocyte called a plasma cell. There are three main types of immunoglobulin called A, G and M. They specifically bind to foreign substances, trying to eliminate them and are then called 'antibodies'.

antibody
A specific immunoglobulin molecule directed against a particular substance (an 'antigen').

autoimmune disease
A disease in which the body's immune system reacts against its own antigens as if they were foreign.

particularly the small intestine, it is necessary to understand what is abnormal in coeliac disease. In Chapter 3 we will explore who gets coeliac disease and why, and how the abnormalities develop. Here, however, it is important to summarize what changes from normal in the coeliac gut.

It is reassuring to know that the major structure of the whole of the gut remains normal in coeliac disease. The total length of the gut, including the small intestine, is not shortened and the four layers of the bowel wall are also intact. The major abnormalities are only in the mucosa of the small intestine.

Mucosal abnormalities

Bearing in mind the mucosal structure in Figure 2.3, in coeliac disease the villi are much shorter and may be absent. The crypts are increased in depth, as is the lamina propria which contains many more immune cells than usual.

In Plate 6 the surface of the coeliac mucosa is seen through a magnifying glass. The villi are absent and one can see the openings into 'vestibules' at the top of the crypts. The mucosa looks 'flat' in appearance, or even has a 'mosaic' pattern.

In Plate 7 we see the histological features of a vertically cut section of a biopsy viewed down a microscope. It is easy to see the lack of villi, the deep crypts and the thick lamina propria which has many more cells than usual.

The epithelial layer of enterocytes shows that the individual cells are no longer the normal rectangular shape, but more cube-like or flattened. In between the enterocytes there are

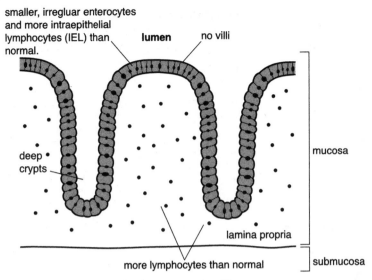

smaller, irregluar enterocytes and more intraepithelial lymphocytes (IEL) than normal.

lumen

no villi

deep crypts

mucosa

lamina propria

more lymphocytes than normal

submucosa

Figure 2.5 Untreated coeliac mucosa showing no villi, deep crypts and more lymphocytes than normal.

more 'intraepithelial' lymphocytes than normal. These changes are seen in Figure 2.5.

These mucosal changes can vary substantially between patients. In some patients there are quite reasonably shaped villi, even though they are shorter than normal; similarly, the crypts may not be severely abnormal in all patients. Why there is a range of severity of mucosal abnormalities in coeliac disease is an ongoing puzzle, which is discussed further in Chapter 5. Not only that, but the extent of the abnormal mucosa down the length of the small intestine also varies, in some affecting much of the small bowel, in others only the duodenum and upper jejunum.

If the enterocytes are examined with the electron microscope, then the microvilli which form the outer surface are also affected. In Plate 8 the microvilli are obviously short and fragmented.

Functional abnormalities

At the functional level, the main effects are as a result of those changes found in the mucosa described above. A poorly functioning mucosa results in poor secretions from the **pancreas** and the bile duct. Consequently, even the early stages of digestion may be affected in coeliac patients.

Obviously the reduction in the villi, with resulting loss of surface area for absorption, means that the final digestive processes at the surface of the cells and the absorption across the epithelium into the bloodstream are severely affected. As described in Chapter 4, this leads to gastrointestinal symptoms in some patients, and nutritional deficiencies in all.

As a consequence of the mal-absorption and mal-digestion, there is more fluid and partially digested food in the intestinal lumen than usual. The coeliac mucosa is also sloughing-off more cells and secreting more immunoglobulins than normal, hence there are excess contents within the intestine which can cause symptoms of wind, bloating, distension, pain and diarrhoea.

The immune system is activated in coeliac disease (see Chapter 3) as evidenced by the increase in the lymphocytes in the lamina propria and epithelium and the increased secretion of immunoglobulin A (IgA), described above.

A final comment in this chapter is to remind the reader that, in the vast majority of coeliac patients, the abnormalities described return to normal on treatment with a gluten-free diet.

pancreas
An organ behind the stomach and close to the duodenum. It produces several chemicals, including insulin which passes into the blood to control the sugar levels. It also produces chemicals into the duodenum which begin the breakdown of food into simpler chemical substances.

Q **What are the vitamins which I may not absorb very well in coeliac disease?**

A There are several vitamins which you may not absorb very well. These include the water-soluble vitamins B, C and folic acid. There are also fat-soluble vitamins which should be borne in mind since fat and fat-soluble vitamins may be particularly poorly absorbed in severe cases. These are vitamins A, D, E and K.

CHAPTER

3

Who gets coeliac disease and how is it caused?

Coeliac disease was originally described in Europe and much of our knowledge about the disease and how to deal with it has grown out of the work of doctors and clinical scientists working in European countries. The reasons for this are most probably based on inherited and environmental factors, like so many diseases. As regards coeliac disease, the European populations, particularly in the northern countries, are very similar genetically and their diets not only have a major dairy component, but are also based on the cereal wheat and the related cereals, rye and barley. The relevance of these factors will become apparent below, when we discuss how coeliac disease is caused.

The frequency of coeliac disease

Reports of the **prevalence** of coeliac disease, that is the number of patients within a given

prevalence
The frequency of something within a given number, for example, the number of cases of a disease within a specific number of the general population. The prevalence of coeliac disease is probably 1 in each 100 people in the general population.

Q Why is coeliac disease more common in populations of European descent?

A There are several possible reasons. A cereal-based diet using wheat has been used traditionally for thousands of years in Northern Europe. There is a common genetic ancestry in European populations. The disease is more often diagnosed since it was first described in Europe and taught about, and there are well-developed health care facilities in many areas where those of European descent have settled.

population, are numerous from European countries and, until recently, it was said that coeliac disease occurred in 1 in 300 to 1 in 1,000 of the population. This was thought to be the case in the UK. However, in the last ten years more reliable blood tests have become available, which give a good indication of whether or not the disease is present. Based on these tests, the prevalence of the disease is now thought to be 1 in 100 of the population. This is so for most European countries where tests have been performed in healthy groups of individuals, for example, blood donors. Of course, many of these people will be undiagnosed and will be unaware that they may have coeliac disease.

Outside Europe there is less information available about the prevalence of coeliac disease but where there are significant populations of people of European ancestry, for example, Australia or South America, the prevalence appears to be similar to that in Europe. Interestingly, the disease has always been said to be rare in the USA, although more recent studies suggest that it has been significantly underestimated. In such a large country, however, with a diverse racial mix in the population with varying dietary traditions, the prevalence of the disease is likely to be variable.

The disease certainly occurs in Asian populations, but will depend upon a wheat-containing diet for it to be evident. There is a significant number of Asian coeliac patients living in European countries, presumably because their diet has become more 'westernized'. The disease, however, is very rare in Chinese or Japanese people. The same is true of African-Caribbean people.

One has to remember that in many developing countries diagnostic facilities are almost non-existent, malnutrition is common and many gastrointestinal symptoms are due to infectious diseases, hence coeliac disease will not be looked for and will not be regarded as a major medical issue.

The coeliac iceberg

As described above, the prevalence figures in Europe now suggest that 1 in 100 of the population may have the disease. However, it is probably the case that only about 1 in 800 of the population is actually diagnosed. This is due to several factors. Many potential patients will have no, or very minor, symptoms; hence they will regard themselves as healthy. The symptoms patients do have can be very diverse (see Chapter 4) and thus it is not always obvious to doctors that coeliac disease may be a cause of the particular symptoms in an individual patient. The severity of symptoms can be variable at different times of life in a patient, and so that might affect which diagnoses might be considered. As described in Chapter 4, there are some trigger factors in a minority of coeliac patients which seem to cause the disease to become symptomatic. Because of the relationship to a wheat-containing diet, the normal diet of an individual may obviously be very relevant to when and how the disease declares itself.

As a result of these factors, and as our understanding of coeliac disease has grown, the concept has arisen of the 'coeliac iceberg', as shown in Figure 3.1. The diagnosed patients are those at the tip of the iceberg, above the

Q Why is coeliac disease less common in some racial groups?

A This is presumed to be partly due to the different genetic inheritance of different races, hence inter-mixing could make the disease more likely in the future. The traditional diet is also important, since wheat and related cereals have to be eaten to precipitate the disease. The disease also has to be diagnosed, which is difficult to do when medical facilities are not so well developed.

Q How common is coeliac disease?

A Surveys of healthy populations in Europe, using a blood test, suggest that 1 person in 100 has coeliac disease. However, probably only 1 in 8 of these has been medically diagnosed with the disease.

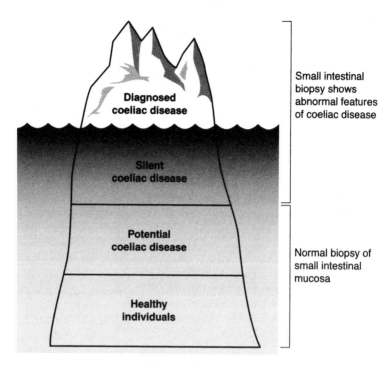

‖ Figure 3.1 The coeliac iceberg.

water-line. These patients will be those with either typical symptoms or more atypical (unusual) features, as described in Chapter 4. They will have an abnormal small intestinal biopsy. The first group below the water-line are the 'silent' coeliac patients. This group will have no symptoms or very few, they will be undiagnosed medically, but a biopsy would show an abnormal small intestine. They may develop symptoms at any time, and some adults may have had symptoms as children. It is also believed they could develop complications of coeliac disease (see Chapter 6), although there is not much evidence for this at present. These patients would have a positive blood test for coeliac disease, if tested.

my experience

As a girl I was well and my mother tells me I only had the usual childhood illnesses. I enjoyed school and had a happy childhood. After starting secondary school, the other girls teased me since I was late in developing and my periods didn't start until I was about 15 years of age. I hated games and was always tired in the evenings. I left school at 16. My mother went with me to the doctor's surgery because of my tiredness, but he said I was still growing and that everything would be all right. He did measure my blood count on one occasion, which showed I was anaemic. He said it was my periods and gave me some iron tablets.

I got a job at a nursery and eventually trained to be a nursery nurse. I met Bob when I was 22 and we have been together ever since. We had our first child when I was 25. The hospital were always checking my blood count during the pregnancy and afterwards. In fact, after the delivery of Beth, I needed a blood transfusion. Kelly was born four years later but, once again, there was a lot of worry about me being anaemic.

Last year we had a party for my fortieth birthday. My sister Jo came from Australia and she had just been diagnosed with coeliac disease. She had a difficult time at the party; we didn't know what we could give her to eat, but fortunately she is pretty smart and knew exactly what to do.

The GP had still been giving me iron tablets from time to time since whenever my blood count was checked I was always anaemic. I told him about my sister and how strange her diet seemed. He suggested I had a blood test for coeliac disease too. Of course, you can guess the outcome. It was positive. Then I had a biopsy test at the local hospital and it showed I also had the disease. Now I've been on a gluten-free diet for six months. It was difficult at first, but once you get the hang of things it's worth it. Funnily enough, I do feel better. I had thought getting over 40 was a bad thing and I was slowing down. Now I am full of energy; the girls think I'm a new woman!

There is, then, a group of patients who may develop the disease but who currently have no symptoms and have a normal small intestinal mucosa. These would probably, however, have a positive blood test. They are a group of healthy individuals who are 'potential' coeliac patients. For obvious reasons, very few have been identified and followed-up for a long time in order to see what happens, since they are only likely to be discovered by chance. However, some such patients, sometimes confusingly called 'latent coeliac patients', have been shown to go on to be diagnosed with typical coeliac disease. All of the above three categories would fall into the 1 in 100 prevalence figure quoted above. Those above the water-line, that is diagnosed patients, would be the 1 in 800. All of these individuals in the three categories would be expected to have a similar genetic make-up, although the detail of that is not yet fully known. However, there are people in the population also with that genetic background and, for reasons not understood, they will not develop coeliac disease; these are the healthy individuals at the base of the iceberg.

Screening for coeliac disease

The advent of quite a specific blood test has enabled more patients to be identified and the prevalence figure of 1 in 100 to be obtained. It raises the question of mass **screening** for coeliac disease. However, there is no universal agreement on this. Clearly, it would be possible to identify many more people by the blood test; they would then need to be diagnosed by a biopsy and a gluten-free diet recommended as appropriate. The expectation would then be that

screening
Testing a healthy population of people for the occurrence of a disease or abnormality.

their long-term health should be improved. However, since such individuals, identified by screening, are by definition 'well', and many remain without symptoms, one has to be sure that making a diagnosis, with the necessary dietary recommendations, is the correct treatment or medical management. There is no good long-term evidence yet that this is so. There is, however, a good case for seeking the disease in those individuals who are more likely to have coeliac disease, for example, those with insulin-dependent diabetes or thyroid disease, or who are close relatives of coeliac patients (see Chapter 4). This is called 'case finding'.

The genetics of coeliac disease

There is an undoubted family tendency to coeliac disease, although this is not very strong. Many coeliac patients do know of a close relative who has the disease. Nevertheless, it is a minority of patients. Several studies have confirmed that approximately 1 in 10 patients will have a first-degree relative with the condition: that is a parent, brother or sister, or child with the disease. This familial tendency is also evident in studies of twins. The prevalence in non-identical twins is similar to that in brothers or sisters, but in at least 70 per cent of identical twin pairs both twins will have the disease. If both twins were observed throughout their whole lives, it is highly likely that the figure would be more than 70 per cent since they can develop symptoms at different ages. This occurrence rate in twins is called 'concordance', thus there is 70 per cent concordance in identical twins for coeliac disease.

> **Q** My husband has had coeliac disease since he was a baby. I am now pregnant with our first child; will he/she have coeliac disease?
>
> **A** There is a 1 in 10 chance of a first-degree relative of a coeliac patient having the disease. A first-degree relative is a parent, a brother or sister, or a child, so your child has a 1 in 10 chance. This risk is not as high as it seems initially. It suggests one out of ten children could develop the disease (if you had ten!). The risk is that you do not know which one and, of course, for every child it is the same risk. The good thing to remember is that you can be aware of the risk and look for any possible developing symptoms as the baby grows.

Specific genetic findings

The genetics of coeliac disease have been studied in more detail by examination of individual **genes**. What is a gene? Technically a gene is a unit of inheritance. We inherit half our genes from each parent. Each gene is a short string of chemicals arranged in a specific order which can be used by the cells of the body to make a particular bodily protein. There are approximately 30,000 human genes. We all have our own individual genes, and copies of all 30,000 are in the nucleus of each of our body's cells. Most work in coeliac disease has been done on some of the genes that are responsible for our 'tissue type', that is the genes which are used for organ matching in transplantation. Many of these genes are also related to our immune system.

It is now known that one of two groups of 'tissue type' genes we call **DQ2** or **DQ8** is present in virtually all coeliac patients. In fact, it is considered most unlikely that an individual without either of those particular genes could have coeliac disease. However, although 100 per

genes
Units of inheritance each made up of a string of chemicals (**DNA**) in the nucleus of each cell of our bodies, which vary from person to person.

DNA (deoxyribose nucleic acid)
The chemical which is used by the body to make up our genes.

DQ2/DQ8
The symbol of two particular tissue types which are inherited via specific genes. They are present in virtually all coeliac patients, but also in about 30 per cent of non-coeliac people.

cent of patients are either DQ2 or DQ8 positive, so are approximately 30 per cent of the rest of the population who do not have coeliac disease. Hence, these particular genes are referred to as *necessary* to have the disease, but not *sufficient*. That is, there must be something else, either genetic or environmental, which is required in those other 30 per cent of people who are DQ2 or DQ8 positive in order to develop coeliac disease.

Mathematical predictions on the genetics of coeliac disease suggest that there are other genes involved. There have been several studies of other genes in coeliac patients, but none have yet been fruitful. Several are still ongoing. For such studies to be reliable, they require samples from hundreds of properly diagnosed patients, and they are very costly to run. Currently we await further results.

 Q I have coeliac disease, does that mean I have a coeliac disease gene?

 A No, this is not the case and it is unlikely that a single gene or defective gene will be found which is solely responsible for the disease. We know that individuals have to have certain genes before they can develop the disease, but most people who have those genes do not develop coeliac disease, so that is not the whole story. No doubt some other genes will be discovered which play a part, but it is highly likely that eventually several genes will be found which interact so that the individual, when exposed to gluten, will develop the disease.

myth
Finding a coeliac disease gene will stigmatize coeliac patients.

fact
Finding a specific set of genes which is causative for coeliac disease is likely to be very helpful in diagnosing and finding new treatments. Coeliac disease is not a disease to be frightened of, and not a risky disease to have. Genetic findings should not stigmatize patients.

How is coeliac disease caused?

It has already been explained that genetic and environmental influences are necessary to have

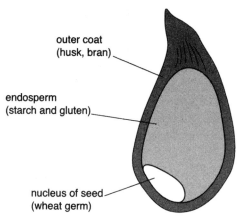

outer coat
(husk, bran)

endosperm
(starch and gluten)

nucleus of seed
(wheat germ)

Figure 3.2 A simplified diagram of a cereal (wheat) seed.

coeliac disease. Some of the genes have been identified, and the main environmental factor has also been known for well over 50 years, that is, the part of wheat and related cereals called gluten.

What is gluten?

Gluten is the storage protein in wheat, rye and barley which provides a nitrogen source for the plant, and also for people when the cereal is part of the diet. The gluten is stored in the seed as shown in Figure 3.2. After the cereal (wheat, rye or barley) is harvested, the milling process results in the removal of the outer coat from the seeds, which leaves the endosperm. This is ground up to produce flour, which is mostly starch (carbohydrate) but also contains the gluten.

If wheat flour is washed in water, starch (the carbohydrate part), together with some minerals, is dissolved out. One is left with a sticky, rubbery mass we call gluten (see Figure 3.3). Gluten is principally a mixture of proteins which have the

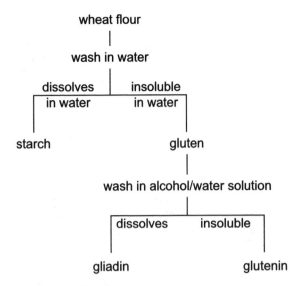

wheat flour
|
wash in water

dissolves in water | insoluble in water

starch

gluten
|
wash in alcohol/water solution

dissolves | insoluble

gliadin

glutenin

▮ Figure 3.3 The parts of wheat flour.

physical properties (cohesivity and visco-elasticity) which are responsible for the unique baking quality of wheat. When cooked, these proteins swell and trap air and form a nice structure to the loaf or cake, giving it a texture which is good to eat. Over thousands of years, farmers have bred wheat of different varieties to improve its baking qualities. This has been good for human nutrition and cooks, but not so good for coeliac patients since modern wheats probably have proportionately more gluten, which triggers coeliac disease in susceptible individuals. This may partly account for the increase in the number of cases.

Gluten has traditionally been studied by cereal chemists who divided it into two 'fractions', **gliadin** and glutenin (see Figure 3.3), gliadin being soluble in a mixture of alcohol and water. Gliadin is a mixture of many similar **proteins** of somewhat different sizes, which vary slightly

gliadin
The part of gluten which is soluble in an alcohol/water solution.

protein
A long run of amino acids joined together which forms a particular structure, for example, tissue fibres, walls of cells, enzymes (proteins which cause chemical reactions). Eating food which contains protein supplies the body with a source of nutrition and energy from the amino acids.

depending upon the type of wheat used to produce the flour. Gliadins have been divided into four groups called α (alpha), β (beta), γ (gamma) and ω (omega) gliadins.

Modern analysis of proteins is now very detailed and for many of the proteins in gluten (both the gliadins and the glutenins) their primary structure is now known.

A protein is made up of a string of **amino acids**, which are the basic chemical building blocks in biology. There are 20 amino acids found in living organisms, and a protein is made up of hundreds or thousands of these joined together in different combinations. This is the primary structure of the protein. The number of each amino acid present and the sequence of them all is controlled and ordered by the genes of the particular organism.

Throughout the evolution of wheat, the wheat genes which determine the primary structure of gliadins and glutenins have been developed in order to produce crops which are more productive and probably nutritious. Different wheat varieties produce slightly different gliadin and glutenin proteins, each of which has different baking qualities. The glutenin proteins are much bigger than the gliadin proteins. For example, a gliadin protein may be 250–300 amino acids in length, whereas a glutenin protein may be 700–800 amino acids long. What is very characteristic about all these proteins is that they have large numbers of two particular amino acids, glutamine and proline.

How do we know gluten is involved in coeliac disease?

Samuel Gee, a physician at St Bartholomew's Hospital in London, wrote the first proper

> **amino acid**
> A basic chemical building block in biology. There are 20 amino acids which are common throughout nature. When they are combined together in various sequences, they form proteins.

description of coeliac disease in 1888. In those days the cause of the disease was not known but he did say that he thought it was due to the diet in some way (see Chapter 1). It was 60 to 70 years later, in the 1950s, when it was found that wheat, and in particular the gluten part of wheat flour, was responsible for precipitating symptoms. These clinical studies over 50 years ago observed groups of patients taking either gluten-containing or gluten-free diets and noting what clinical effects and symptoms the presence or absence of gluten in the diet produced.

As time went on, our understanding of the make-up of the gluten proteins developed, as did our means of studying the intestinal mucosa and the immune mechanisms of the body. In the 1970s and 1980s a technique was developed for maintaining small intestinal mucosal biopsies alive in the laboratory for several days. Different small fragments of gluten proteins could be added in the nutrient fluid around these biopsies, and the effects of these fragments measured. This has been an immensely useful technique for studying coeliac disease. For example, I was able to show that samples of α-, β-, γ- and ω-gliadin from one strain of wheat were all capable of damaging coeliac mucosa in this test system, although there was a graded effect, α-gliadin being the worst and ω-gliadin the least damaging.

Nowadays, it is possible to separate out immune cells (lymphocytes) from mucosal biopsies and also from blood samples of coeliac patients. These lymphocytes can be tested against gluten fragments in the laboratory. Coeliac lymphocytes are much more sensitive to such fragments than lymphocytes from non-coeliac patients. In such test systems, which are very sensitive, it is possible to predict which fragments of gluten may be causally involved in coeliac disease.

We have already noted that proteins are long chains of amino acids. A short length containing a small number of amino acids is called a **peptide**. Researchers in coeliac disease are now testing peptides of approximately 20 amino acids long in the lymphocyte and biopsy test systems described above. In these peptides the amino acids glutamine and proline are frequently repeated. So, the particular fragments of gluten, and thus wheat flour, which may cause coeliac disease are slowly being discovered. Theoretically, a wheat free of the specific coeliac-causing peptides would be safe for coeliac patients to eat. However, it is important to note that these short peptides are frequently repeated throughout the different gliadins and glutenins which make up the various glutens of different wheats, therefore it will not be easy to produce wheat so that its flour is without them and, even if possible, its baking properties may not be good.

Another important point to remember is that although significant advances in our understanding of the cause of coeliac disease have been made using laboratory tests, ultimately any new dietary change has to be tested in patients over time for its safety. There are a few scientific studies where patients have valiantly volunteered to have biopsy tests before and after taking gluten peptides to see if they have any detrimental effect.

> **peptide**
> A short run of amino acids joined together.

Wheat and related cereals

To complete the description of wheat gluten, we should note the relationships with other cereals. In Figure 3.4 we see the family relationships of some of the various grasses in botany.

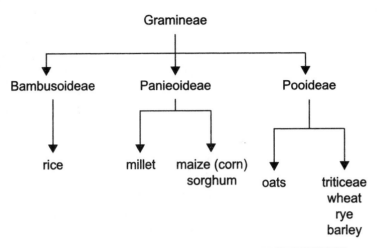

Figure 3.4 Branches of the different cereals in the grass family.

It can be seen that the family 'triticeae' contains three related cereals (wheat, rye, barley), all of which are implicated in the causation of coeliac disease. Oats is a 'near cousin', but is now believed to be safe for coeliac patients (see Chapter 6). It can be seen that rice and maize (corn) are only distant relatives, with very different proteins in their make-up, and thus are safe for coeliac patients to eat.

Rye and barley can be studied in a similar way to wheat. The gluten in rye is called **secalin** and that of barley is called **hordein**. These proteins, however, are all very similar in amino acid primary structure and there is no doubt that rye and barley are just as much implicated in coeliac disease as wheat.

How does gluten cause the mucosal abnormality characteristic of coeliac disease?

Once it was found out that the gluten proteins in wheat (and closely related cereals) were

secalin
The name for the gluten equivalent in rye.

hordein
The name for the gluten equivalent in barley.

myth
Gluten occurs only in wheat.

fact
Scientifically, gluten is the word for that particular protein mixture which occurs in wheat. However, there are very similar protein mixtures in rye and barley which, scientifically, are called secalin and hordein respectively. Because they are all closely related chemicals, and all cause the coeliac abnormality in susceptible individuals, the shorthand term 'gluten' is used to cover them all.

fact
There is no evidence for this whatsoever. Scientists have sometimes wondered whether an infection in the intestine could start the disease off, but even then there is virtually no scientific evidence for this at present.

responsible for precipitating coeliac disease, work began to understand how. Several theories were initially suggested, but it is now established that the underlying mechanism is immunological. The study of coeliac disease itself has been very instrumental in furthering our understanding of the immune system of the intestine, so medical researchers are very grateful to all those patients who have allowed blood samples and mucosal biopsies to be used in medical research.

In Chapter 2 a description was given of the immune system in the mucosa of the small intestine. Essentially, the basic immune reaction believed to underline coeliac disease is as follows (see Figure 3.5).

The gluten peptides pass across the epithelium of the small intestine into the lamina propria part of the mucosa. They come into contact with an enzyme, tissue transglutaminase, which slightly modifies the gluten peptide. These peptides are then taken into special cells (antigen-presenting cells) and put onto the surface of those cells in combination with the 'tissue type' molecules (DQ2/DQ8, see section on genetics above). This makes the gluten peptide able to be recognized as an antigen by the lymphocytes. The lymphocytes are then activated and they multiply rapidly and, although spreading throughout the body, they concentrate in the small intestinal mucosa, being attracted to the gluten peptides. They produce immune chemicals, including immunoglobulins (antibodies). Inflammation of the mucosa results as more lymphocytes are produced. This is a typical immune reaction and is aimed at eliminating the 'foreign' gluten but, of course, also damages the mucosa and thus causes the abnormalities seen in coeliac disease:

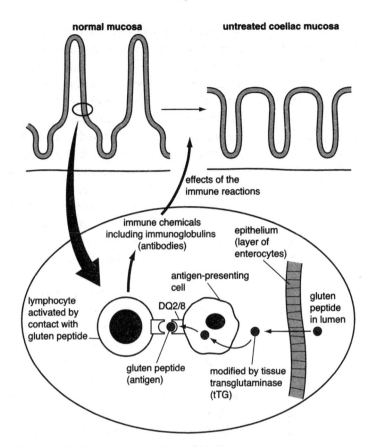

Figure 3.5 The immune reaction in the small intestinal mucosa against gluten produces the coeliac abnormality.

a decrease in the height of the villi and an increase in the depth of the crypts (Figure 3.5). Elimination of gluten from the diet allows this immune reaction to cease and the mucosa to return to normal. Since the immune reaction is not only against gluten but against the body itself, thus coeliac disease is often referred to as an autoimmune disease.

myth
Coeliac disease is like any other food allergy.

fact
Coeliac disease is a condition where there is a definite abnormality in the intestine which can be related causally to gluten in the diet. The abnormality is immunologically produced, but it is not a typical 'allergy' like the reaction some people have to nuts, or the asthma provoked by pollen. In the vast majority of cases of food allergy there is no abnormality to be demonstrated in the intestine. Although food intolerances or allergies do exist, they should not be confused with coeliac disease.

CHAPTER

4 How does coeliac disease affect the patient?

As described in Chapters 2 and 3, the small intestine becomes abnormal in coeliac disease and this results in a number of clinical features. There may be gastrointestinal symptoms due to the abnormal gut. More general symptoms may also develop as a result of poor absorption of dietary nutrients by the abnormal gut and the underlying autoimmune nature of coeliac disease, leading to some systemic clinical problems, i.e. problems affecting other parts of the body.

It is obvious from this that people with coeliac disease can have a wide variety of clinical features of very varying severity. Why people vary so much in their symptoms is unknown. Those patients who have predominantly gastrointestinal symptoms are said to have 'classical' coeliac disease; those who have more general, mainly non-gastrointestinal symptoms are said to have 'atypical' coeliac disease, and those with no

> **myth**
> Coeliac disease occurs only in children.

> **fact**
> Coeliac disease can cause a clinical problem at any age and doctors should always bear it in mind in children or adults when appropriate. The initial reports were often in children who had severe symptoms, hence the myth developed that it is a children's disease.

symptoms have 'silent' coeliac disease. All the patients would have a characteristic intestinal abnormality on biopsy. Coeliac disease can produce clinical effects at any age but there are two peaks of incidence, one in early childhood and the other in middle age (see Figure 4.1).

Coeliac disease in childhood

Approximately 30 per cent of all patients who are eventually diagnosed with coeliac disease will have had symptoms attributable to the disease in childhood. Not all of these, however, will have had a diagnosis made as children.

The majority of children who are diagnosed develop quite marked symptoms early in life, between six months and two years of age. Boys and girls are equally affected. Symptoms develop only after weaning, at between six and nine months, when they are established on a diet containing cereals, especially wheat. There is some evidence that the longer the breast feeding and the later the introduction of cereals takes place, the later the onset of symptoms or there

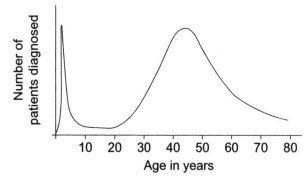

Figure 4.1 Ages at diagnosis of coeliac disease. There are two peaks – in infants and in middle age.

may even be prevention of coeliac symptoms developing. The affected infants may develop quite severe diarrhoea, vomiting and a swollen abdomen, and are generally unwell and miserable (see Plate 9). It is often in marked contrast to their initial progress. They stop putting on weight and look malnourished. Their muscles can become wasted and 'floppy'; this is called hypotonia. Children with these symptoms are being diagnosed earlier as greater awareness of coeliac disease develops, and hence severely affected children should become less common.

my experience

Emma was born at the local hospital. She was our first child and the pregnancy had gone surprisingly well. Everything was OK and we went home within 24 hours. I was very concerned, however, about the breast feeding since there is so much publicity about how important it is. My mother and sisters live at the other end of the country and I wasn't sure who I would turn to for help.

Emma was a restless child, particularly compared with Thomas who was born two years later. She didn't sleep well and the breast feeding didn't go well either. I soon had to supplement that with bottle feeding – it seemed the only way to settle her, particularly in the evenings. I gave up all attempts at breast feeding after two months, after an attack of mastitis and started her on solids soon after. Emma seemed to grow all right but, by six months, I thought something was definitely wrong. She seemed much less lively than other babies, she had a lot of vomiting and diarrhoea on and off, and when she was weighed at the clinic the nurse said she was almost 'off the graph'. That really made me panic.

We asked to see the local specialist and got an appointment quite quickly. He thought that she was probably not getting enough to eat because of the vomiting, and agreed she was small. He suggested she might be allergic to cow's milk or even have cystic fibrosis. He tried to be reassuring, but you can imagine the panic. He arranged some tests and suggested we started using soya milk. Nigel got on the internet as soon as we got home. That made us even more worried.

Changing the diet didn't help, and the tests for cystic fibrosis were normal. However, the specialist had also sent a blood test for coeliac disease and this proved to be positive. He suggested a biopsy test via the endoscopy camera test, which would need an anaesthetic. We agreed to that and Emma had it the following week. The biopsy showed typical coeliac disease and a gluten-free diet was recommended. Within two to three weeks we saw a difference. She became more lively and there was no more vomiting; her stools soon became much more normal and nowadays she is more constipated if anything. During the four to six months after starting the diet, her weight increased quite dramatically and she is now in the centre of the graph.

We have learned to cope with a gluten-free diet and Emma knows no different. She is now a happy three-year-old child. My only worry now is about whether Thomas may have coeliac disease, but he is growing well with no medical problems, so I shall just wait and see for the time being.

Some children develop symptoms in later childhood, between the ages of two and ten. In these children there are more minor gastrointestinal symptoms, perhaps recurrent stomach pains or swelling, intermittent diarrhoea or even constipation. The children may be shorter than expected, with delayed growth or delayed puberty and may have been thought to have a hormonal cause for this. Developmental abnormalities of the enamel on teeth have been described. The children may be lacking in energy and vitality, and have behavioural or learning difficulties. Some children will be found to have **anaemia** or, rarely, to have other nutritional problems, such as rickets.

Plotting children's growth charts shows how their weight and height can be observed over time, and can certainly show the effects of treatment with a gluten-free diet (see Figure 4.2). Some children are now being identified for coeliac disease by screening with a blood test, perhaps because of a family history of the disease. Although these children may be well, with no symptoms, a recent survey which screened several thousand seven-year-old school children found that those with a positive screening test were, on average, slightly shorter and lighter. This suggests that undiagnosed coeliac disease with no obvious symptoms can still lead to a small but significant effect on growth.

Rarely, coeliac disease in children can be associated with other conditions, such as insulin-dependent **diabetes** or Down's syndrome.

Some children with these conditions are now screened for coeliac disease using the blood test once every one to two years, since a negative blood test may become positive over time if the disease is developing. Some of these associations, which occur more in adults, are described later in this chapter. Children, as opposed to adults, are more likely, especially as infants, to have other food intolerances, such as to cow's milk, rice, soya and eggs. Such intolerances can cause confusion with coeliac disease and should be carefully assessed by medical specialists.

anaemia
This is present when there is a reduced level of haemoglobin. Haemoglobin is the red chemical in the red blood cells, which carries oxygen to all parts of the body.

diabetes
This is a disease in which there is a high blood sugar level due to a reduction of, or lack of response to, the hormone insulin from the pancreas. Type 1 diabetes usually occurs in younger people and they require insulin injections for treatment. Type 2 occurs in older, often overweight, people and usually can be treated with tablets.

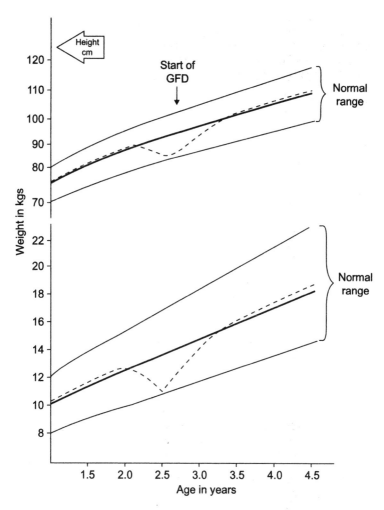

Figure 4.2 Typical growth chart of a child diagnosed with coeliac disease at age two-and-a-half. The normal weight gain tails off prior to diagnosis but picks up well following the introduction of a gluten-free diet. The growth in height shows this less, but there is still an effect.

Q **I was diagnosed with coeliac disease last year and am now feeling much better. I have two children, aged four and two years of age. Should they be tested for coeliac disease?**

A This is difficult to answer categorically. If your children are unwell or not developing properly, your doctor should certainly be aware that you have coeliac disease and this should be a prompt to look for it in your children. If you think your children have coeliac disease, it is better not to stop gluten. Carry on with a normal (gluten-containing) diet until a diagnosis is made. If, however, they are perfectly well with no medical problems, it is probably better not to screen for coeliac disease at present. It should always be borne in mind, however, when medical issues are being raised. Testing does include a blood test, so you would probably only want to consider a screening test if a blood sample was being taken for another necessary medical investigation.

myth
Children grow out of it.

fact
If correctly diagnosed, coeliac disease is a life-long disease. However, it is known that the sensitivity to the effect of gluten varies between individuals and also throughout life in the same individual. Hence, some children appear to get better, and when they are older children or teenagers can eat a normal diet with no symptoms. Such patients are likely to develop symptoms later, and if a biopsy were taken they would probably have an abnormality in the intestine. That is why a gluten-free diet is always recommended for life, even if they have no symptoms.
Children and teenagers with coeliac disease on a gluten-free diet are healthy, grow normally and can do everything that their friends can.

Coeliac disease in teenagers

Some teenagers have few symptoms due to coeliac disease, even those who have been diagnosed as young children. Obviously, these patients should be taking a gluten-free diet, but teenagers often find this difficult. Interestingly, even though they may be taking significant amounts of gluten in their diet, few will have true coeliac symptoms. It is well recognized that an individual's sensitivity to gluten appears to vary at different times during life, and some teenagers are able to take significant amounts of gluten with no apparent ill-effects. This does not mean they should relax their diet. When they go back to a gluten-free diet they often realize that they were not quite right, perhaps a bit tired, when they were cheating.

Teenagers do find the gluten-free diet difficult, since they do not want to be different from their friends and peer pressure is very great to eat popular teenage food which may contain a lot of gluten. This is, of course, reinforced by the finding that gluten may not produce any symptoms and they question whether or not they do have coeliac disease. Indeed, in past times, paediatricians often believed that children 'grew out of' coeliac disease. It is now known that coeliac disease is a life-long condition even if the sensitivity to gluten, and therefore the clinical symptoms, varies throughout life.

The teenager's ability to eat a bit of gluten without significant symptoms is the reason why very few patients are newly diagnosed as teenagers. There will, of course, be a small number of older children, perhaps with delayed development, who are diagnosed as teenagers when the diagnosis has only just become apparent or been considered a possibility. Thinning of the bones (**osteoporosis**), although common in adults with coeliac disease, can occur

---

Q I have recently been diagnosed with coeliac disease, and although I understand the gluten-free diet, I do not like it. If I stick to it until my biopsy improves, will I then be cured?

A If coeliac disease has been properly diagnosed, there is no cure in the sense that it gets better and the patient can then eat a normal diet – 'Once a coeliac, always a coeliac.' However, sticking to a gluten-free diet should return the patient to normal health. If you are struggling with the diet, help is available (see Chapter 7).

---

osteoporosis

A progressive disease of all the bones in which they become less dense and therefore weakened. There is a resulting increased risk of fracture.

in teenagers with the disease. Teenagers should be encouraged to keep in touch with medical care despite their busy lifestyles, even if they refuse to take a strict gluten-free diet, so that any new problems or questions can be discussed.

Coeliac disease in adults

The range of medical problems which cause coeliac disease to be diagnosed in adults has changed considerably in the last 25 years. In the past, such patients went to their doctors with marked gastrointestinal or nutritional symptoms, such as diarrhoea and major weight loss. Nowadays, however, the majority of patients have few symptoms and are often diagnosed because of anaemia, or an incidental deficiency on a blood test. This is not necessarily because the disease is becoming less severe, but partly because the medical profession has become more aware of the disease and it is being diagnosed earlier. There are, sadly of course, still cases where, for a variety of reasons, it takes a long time to make the diagnosis. Worldwide, there is still an average of ten years between the onset of symptoms and the diagnosis being made. This is partly due to the wide variety of symptoms and their varying severity in individual patients. The changes in presenting symptoms over recent decades are shown in Figure 4.3.

As already suggested, the peak age for diagnosing coeliac disease in adults is middle age, 40 to 55 years, although it can be diagnosed at any age. More and more patients over 65 years of age are being diagnosed for the first time. These patients often have very few symptoms, although they may have been 'under par' for a

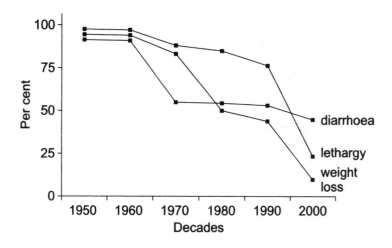

Figure 4.3 Percentages of patients with traditional symptoms at diagnosis. Nowadays the previously universal symptoms of diarrhoea, lethargy and weight loss are much less common at diagnosis.

long time. The ratio of diagnosed female to male adult patients is 2:1.

Approximately 30 per cent of adult patients have a history of symptoms in childhood attributable to coeliac disease, even if it was not then formally diagnosed. In ten per cent of cases there is a family history of the disease, and this may be a reason why some people come to medical attention seeking a diagnosis.

Obviously the main abnormality in coeliac disease is in the intestinal tract, therefore symptoms of diarrhoea, abdominal discomfort, abdominal swelling, indigestion, nausea, vomiting and mouth ulcers occur. As indicated, these 'classical symptoms' used to be seen more frequently in the past when patients were diagnosed much later. Nowadays, the majority of patients have no gastrointestinal symptoms to complain of although, on reflection, once the diagnosis of coeliac disease has been made, some realize they do feel better on treatment and that various abdominal symptoms they regarded as normal were, in fact, indicators of the disease. At least five per cent of patients diagnosed as having the **irritable bowel syndrome** turn out to have coeliac disease. Some patients do lose weight and this also used to be much more common, but nowadays at least 30 per cent of patients are overweight when first diagnosed with coeliac disease.

It has to be stressed, however, that patients with these gastrointestinal related symptoms are in a minority. More patients have atypical, i.e. non-gastrointestinal, symptoms or even no symptoms at all, i.e. silent coeliac disease. These latter patients are diagnosed because of a family history, a positive screening test or a nutritional deficiency.

Patients with atypical symptoms may feel run down or lacking in energy. They may find it difficult to cope with daily activities. Some of the symptoms may be due to anaemia or other nutritional deficiencies, such as low vitamin or mineral levels. Chronic symptoms, particularly with no diagnosis, can obviously lead to depression and anxiety.

Symptoms of joint or muscle pain, unsteadiness of gait (ataxia), and changes in skin sensation due to disturbed nerve function (peripheral neuropathy), can occur. Such 'non-specific' symptoms can obviously cause difficulties and delay in making a diagnosis of a disease of the intestine. Patients may have been thought to have arthritis or rheumatism with no definite diagnosis being made. The neurological symptoms of ataxia and peripheral neuropathy,

irritable bowel syndrome (IBS)
A condition in which the bowel habit is erratic and associated with varying degrees of abdominal pain and often bloating but without any recognizable other disease.

myth
Only women get
osteoporosis.

fact
Women and men can get osteoporosis. Everyone's bones get less dense to some degree as they get older. However, bone health is dependent on hormone levels and after the menopause these change significantly in women, leading to a more rapid effect on the bones; hence osteoporosis is more common in post-menopausal women.

DEXA scan
A type of X-ray scanning which measures the density of the bones.

whilst very rare in coeliac disease, are increasingly being recognized.

One longstanding effect of bowel disease is on the bones. These become less dense than usual and eventually osteoporosis can develop. It is often routine nowadays for this to be considered and treated in coeliac disease (see Chapter 6). However, if patients diagnosed with osteoporosis are investigated, between five and ten per cent will be found to have undiagnosed coeliac disease.

Q **I have been diagnosed with coeliac disease and I have heard that one effect is osteoporosis. Do I need a scan for this?**

A Most older teenagers and adults should have a scan to measure the bone mineral density *(DEXA scan)* at around the time of diagnosis, although it has to be said, that there is not universal medical agreement about this. If this scan is normal, a further scan after the menopause in women, and after 55 years of age in men, is recommended. If there is an abnormal scan, appropriate treatment is suggested and follow-up scans after a reasonable length of time may be necessary. Treatment may include calcium and vitamin D tablets, and other medication to strengthen the bones. Regular exercise and stopping smoking are very important to improve the health of bones. Changes in the bones occur slowly, so DEXA scans only every two to three years for follow-up are to be expected.

Problems with fertility also occur in untreated coeliac disease. Adolescent girls, with delayed development due to unrecognized coeliac disease, will obviously have late puberty and late menstrual periods. Malnourished women with a chronic, untreated disease often have scanty or irregular periods and the menopause may occur earlier than expected. In such situations, conception is less likely. Now that the disease is being diagnosed earlier, and is being treated, one would expect fertility to improve. A well-treated coeliac female will have normal hormonal function. A very recent British study confirmed this, in that the fertility of coeliac women compared to the general population was found not to be reduced, although coeliac women did have their children at a slightly later age on average. This, of course, could be due to several reasons. Interestingly, male coeliac patients also have a slightly reduced fertility, which is unexplained, but this does not usually interfere with having a family. Untreated female coeliac patients who become pregnant have an increased risk of miscarriage and, on average, have smaller babies.

Table 1 lists some of the classical and atypical clinical features or reasons which cause patients to be diagnosed with coeliac disease. Severely affected patients may be obviously thin and malnourished, perhaps with a swollen abdomen, swollen legs and weak muscles (see Plate 10). Nowadays these findings would be very rare.

myth
Coeliac disease can be cured by a period of treatment with a gluten-free diet.

fact
The vast majority of patients improve and return to normal with a gluten-free diet. Because of the variability between patients to the effects of gluten, some patients can take gluten with no apparent ill-effects. Once well, therefore, they think they can return to a normal diet. Eventually all patients will redevelop an abnormality of the intestine if they take gluten and clinical effects will result in the long term.
Patients are therefore never 'cured', even though they can feel perfectly well with dietary treatment.

Table 1 Classical and atypical clinical features

Classical	Atypical
Diarrhoea	Anaemia
Abdominal discomfort	Vitamin deficiency
Abdominal swelling	Osteoporosis
Weight loss	Arthritis/rheumatism
Indigestion	Unsteadiness (ataxia)
Mouth ulcers	Changes in skin sensation
Nausea	(peripheral neuropathy)
Vomiting	Reduced fertility
Irritable bowel syndrome	Obesity
Delayed development	Depression/anxiety
Childhood history	Relative with coeliac disease
suggesting coeliac	
disease	

When most new patients with coeliac disease are examined by a doctor, there are very few abnormalities of the body to be found in those patients who have virtually no, or non-specific, symptoms.

Trigger events

As described in Chapter 3, the coeliac abnormality occurs in genetically predisposed individuals in response to eating food containing gluten. One might expect it always to cause symptoms in children soon after the time of weaning when they begin to eat wheat products. Clearly, this is not the case. It is not known why patients present with symptoms for the first time at different ages from infancy to the elderly, even though there are two peaks of age when patients are more likely to be diagnosed. No known trigger factor is obvious in the majority of patients.

There are, however, some known trigger events which, in a few patients, do seem to provoke symptoms and lead them to seek a diagnosis. Following a bout of **gastroenteritis**, often associated with foreign travel, a patient's symptoms may fail to resolve as expected. Coeliac disease is found to be present, even though previously the patient had had no symptoms. Similarly, following surgery, often gastrointestinal surgery, when presumably the normal structure and function of the gut is disturbed or permanently altered, continuing or newly developed symptoms lead to the diagnosis of coeliac disease. Symptoms can develop for the first time during or following pregnancy, leading to the diagnosis in up to 17 per cent of female coeliac patients. Other

gastroenteritis
Usually due to an infection with a bacterium or virus from poorly cooked food or contaminated water. It results in vomiting and diarrhoea. Usually resolves without treatment. If a causative bacterium is cultured from the stool, specific antibiotics may be indicated.

episodes of major stress in a person's life have also been described as precipitating symptoms for the first time. Rarely, coeliac disease is first diagnosed when only one of its complications develops (see Chapter 6).

Clearly, consumption of gluten is necessary for the disease to manifest itself, and hence the amount of wheat and related cereals which is eaten is relevant to the development and diagnosis of coeliac disease. The trigger events are summarized below:

◇ amount of gluten consumed
◇ gastroenteritis (especially associated with foreign travel)
◇ gastrointestinal surgery
◇ pregnancy
◇ stress
◇ complications of coeliac disease.

Associated diseases

Autoimmune diseases

In Chapter 3 the immunological disturbances in coeliac disease were described and it was suggested that the disease could be regarded as an autoimmune disease. There is a group of autoimmune diseases which occur in people who probably have an inherited predisposition to develop them, possibly because they have a genetically more 'sensitive' immune system. Hence, if a patient has one such disease there is an increased risk of developing another one. Three per cent of the general population have an autoimmune disease, but this increases to 30 per cent in coeliac patients, that is coeliac patients are ten times more likely to have another autoimmune

Table 2 Associated autoimmune conditions

Type 1 (insulin-dependent) diabetes mellitus
Autoimmune thyroid disease
Autoimmune liver disease (hepatitis or primary biliary
    cirrhosis)
Autoimmune adrenal disease (Addison's disease)
Inflammatory bowel disease (Crohn's disease, ulcerative
    colitis or lymphocytic colitis)
Parathyroid disorders
Sjögren's syndrome and other connective tissue
    disorders
Pulmonary fibrosis
Cardiac muscle dysfunction (cardiomyopathy)
Immunoglobulin A (IgA) deficiency

disease. The autoimmune disorders which have been described in association with coeliac disease are shown in Table 2. (A description of some of these disorders is beyond the scope of this book.) The previous diagnosis of an autoimmune disease may raise the possibility of coeliac disease, which is then found on investigation. In such a situation, the coeliac symptoms are often very mild (i.e. silent coeliac disease).

The most commonly encountered are insulin-dependent diabetes (Type 1 diabetes) and **thyroid disorders**, which can be either over-activity or under-activity. These two disorders occur in approximately five to eight per cent of coeliac patients and therefore should be borne in mind during follow-up of patients, or when new symptoms develop. The other diseases are rarer and coeliac patients should not expect that they will also develop one of these.

Another immune abnormality which is more common in coeliac patients than in general (one in 40 compared with one in 400) is immunoglobulin A deficiency. This deficiency makes people slightly more prone to respiratory

thyroid disorders
The thyroid gland in the neck produces the hormone thyroxine. Over-production causes excess activity of various bodily functions, leading to weight loss, hyperactivity, 'staring' eyes and anxiety. Under-production causes weight gain, slowing down, and feeling cold.

and gastrointestinal infections but, in practical terms, these are only minor problems and frequently go unnoticed. What is more important is the misleading effect of this deficiency on the antibody tests for coeliac disease (see Chapter 5).

Dermatitis herpetiformis (DH)

This is a rare skin disease and is most common in white European people but in the UK occurs in approximately only one per 10,000 of the population. It usually starts in early adult life, although it can occur at any age, but is very rare in children. It is strongly associated with coeliac disease. Five per cent of patients with coeliac disease are likely to have DH, whereas almost all patients with DH will have an intestinal abnormality similar to that in coeliac disease.

DH causes the skin to form blisters. These start as small red patches, which rapidly develop into intensely itchy blisters. Rupture of the blisters by scratching gives relief and then the scabs heal. The whole process takes seven to ten days. This blistering rash typically occurs symmetrically on the elbows and forearms, the buttocks, knees, shoulders, face, neck and trunk. The rash may be widespread or limited to one or two of these sites. It can occur at sites of pressure or trauma from tight clothing. Without treatment it becomes a persistent disorder and only ten to 15 per cent of patients get better spontaneously.

Associated intestinal abnormality

An important advance was made in the understanding of DH in the 1960s, when it was found that more than 90 per cent of patients with

dermatitis herpetiformis (DH)
A skin condition which has itchy blisters typically on the arms, buttocks and knees. Patients almost all have the small intestinal abnormality of coeliac disease.

DH had a similar mucosal abnormality in the small intestine to that of coeliac disease. In fact, even in the remaining ten per cent of patients there are minor abnormalities in the gut, highly suggestive of those in coeliac disease. Despite these findings, only a few DH patients have bowel symptoms, and only rarely are these severe. It is believed that this is because the gut abnormalities are mild, limited to a short length of the small intestine, and that there is sufficient normal intestine to compensate.

Diagnosis of DH

The correct diagnosis of DH requires a skin biopsy which is taken from normal (uninvolved) skin. The biopsy undergoes special testing for IgA deposits which are diagnostic of DH. All diagnosed patients should have a small intestinal biopsy as do coeliac patients in order to assess the mucosa for the coeliac-like abnormalities (see Chapter 5). As in coeliac disease, antibody tests and assessment for anaemia and nutritional factors should be carried out (see Chapter 5).

Treatment of DH

dapsone
A frequently used medication for dermatitis herpetiformis.

Drug treatment is available for the DH rash and acts quickly and effectively. **Dapsone** is usually the medication tried first. The dose is reduced with the clearance of the rash once it has come under control. Sulphapyridine and sulphamethoxypyridazine are two other effective drugs. All these drugs have side-effects which require medical supervision, but once a drug has been successfully established this can be used in the long term to control the disease.

Of great interest and importance is the dietary treatment. This is identical to that for coeliac disease (see Chapter 6). In DH patients not only the abnormality in the intestine but also the rash responds to a gluten-free diet. Hence, once a gluten-free diet is established, many patients can cease taking the drug treatment, or at least take a very reduced dose. A gluten-free diet is thus strongly recommended in DH, although if drug treatment alone is effective and there are no gut symptoms, patients may find it difficult to accept the need for a diet which is somewhat restricting.

Q My DH rash is well controlled with dapsone; why should I take a gluten-free diet?

A The vast majority of people who have DH also have an abnormality of the small intestine on biopsy, like coeliac patients. Usually, however, this abnormality is not very severe, but it will improve on a gluten-free diet. If you have not already had a biopsy (which must be done while taking a *normal* diet) it is worth discussing the possibility with your doctor. The medical recommendation would be to take a gluten-free diet in order to heal any small intestinal mucosal abnormality, which should make your body healthier. This diet should also help the rash of DH. It may be that you could then stop the dapsone. Dapsone, unfortunately, has no healing effect on the small intestine. Occasionally, dapsone does have side-effects, so these may be avoided. A gluten-free diet also reduces the very small risk of any complications of coeliac disease. Overall, my advice would be to take a gluten-free diet especially if you have an abnormal biopsy.

Association of DH with coeliac disease

As already described, almost all DH patients have an abnormal small intestinal mucosa of varying degree, which is identical to that of coeliac disease. This responds to a gluten-free diet, as does coeliac disease. Essentially, therefore, DH patients have coeliac disease. This is supported by the fact that both diseases have a similar genetic inheritance, and they tend to run in families where some relatives may have DH and others coeliac disease. Identical twins have even been described where one has DH and the other coeliac disease. About five per cent of coeliac patients have DH.

Both are associated with the same range of autoimmune diseases, and both develop the same complications (see Chapter 6). Why patients with a coeliac small intestinal abnormality develop the skin rash of DH is not understood. It is clearly gluten-dependent, so it is presumed that there is an underlying immunological mechanism involving gluten and affecting both the gut and the skin in DH.

CHAPTER

5

How is coeliac disease diagnosed?

A clinical suspicion of coeliac disease

In Chapter 4 we have just seen that patients with coeliac disease can have a wide variety of symptoms, with varying severity, and can be of any age. Not surprisingly, this can lead to puzzlement for the doctor who is trying to decide what the symptoms may be due to, and therefore a delay in diagnosis. It is hoped that raising awareness amongst health care professionals and the general public will improve matters and lead to more prompt diagnosis. The work of patients' societies, such as Coeliac UK, is important in this.

When a patient consults a doctor, therefore, there needs to be a 'high index of suspicion' for coeliac disease, that is, doctors always need to bear in mind the possibility of the disease. Obviously, the presence of gastrointestinal symptoms is a good clue, but we know that these are now less frequently encountered in newly diagnosed patients than previously. Many patients may be overweight, contrary to the traditional teaching that coeliac patients have significant weight loss and gross malnutrition. Nowadays, the patient is most commonly diagnosed because of the findings on a routine blood test.

Routine blood tests

The diagnosis may be suggested because of finding anaemia in a routine blood test. Not only may the patient be anaemic, that is with a reduced haemoglobin level, but the red blood cells may be found to be abnormal. For example, they may be bigger or smaller than normal, suggesting either **folic acid** deficiency or iron deficiency respectively. Such deficiencies may occur due to poor absorption from the small intestine, which can occur in coeliac disease. Because of such features in the red cells, the blood may have been tested for the levels of folic acid, iron or **Vitamin B$_{12}$**, which can also cause bigger cells if low. Apart from a change in the size of the red blood cells, they can have an unusual shape or appearance under the microscope which may suggest that the **spleen** is not working too well, an abnormality which occurs, although rarely, in coeliac disease.

folic acid
An essential vitamin for the body's cells to work properly. Deficiency can particularly cause anaemia. Good sources include liver and green vegetables.

Vitamin B$_{12}$
An essential vitamin for the body's cells to work properly. Deficiency can cause anaemia and nerve damage. Good sources include liver, meat and milk.

spleen
An organ in the left-hand side of the upper abdomen beneath the ribs. It is part of the immune system and helps to develop and store lymphocytes. It also removes and breaks down old cells in the circulating blood. People usually lead normal healthy lives if their spleen has to be removed for any reason.

Q **Why does coeliac disease cause anaemia?**

A The main reason why anaemia occurs in coeliac patients is because in the small intestine the mucosa is damaged and the villi are short or absent. This vastly reduces the surface area for the intestine to absorb food constituents, and anaemia results from the reduced absorption of iron, or folic acid or both despite normal amounts in the diet. More rarely, Vitamin B_{12} absorption is also reduced, which contributes to anaemia. These are often given as supplements, but once coeliac disease is effectively treated their absorption from the diet will be back to normal. Very rarely, in severely ill patients who are untreated, their food intake is very low and they will not be taking enough nutrients in their diet; this will also lead to anaemia.

myth
All people with anaemia have coeliac disease.

fact
There are many causes of anaemia. Some are much more common than coeliac disease. Hence anyone with anaemia must have a proper diagnosis made of its cause.

Other findings on routine blood tests include a low calcium level due to poor absorption, and which might indicate that there is some associated bone disease. A reduced **albumin** level may also occur, indicating excess loss from an abnormal gut or reduced production in a mildly inflamed liver, both of which can occur in coeliac disease. Abnormal liver function is also suggested by a modest rise in the blood level of other chemicals coming from the liver. If the immunoglobulins have been measured and a reduced level of immunoglobulin A (IgA) is found, this may suggest coeliac disease since this deficiency is ten times more common in coeliac patients than normal. Tests of how well the blood clots are may also be mildly abnormal, with an increased clotting time, suggesting Vitamin K deficiency due to its poor absorption from a coeliac intestine. Vitamin K is a necessary vitamin to enable the blood to clot properly.

albumin
A protein in the blood made by the liver.

It can be seen, therefore, that if a number of routine blood tests are performed, one or more abnormalities could be accounted for by the presence of coeliac disease. However, there are several other causes for these abnormalities, some of which are much more common than coeliac disease. Hence, abnormalities in routine blood tests may raise the suspicion of coeliac disease, but need to be interpreted by an astute physician.

More specific blood tests for coeliac disease

In Chapter 3 reference was made to the possibility of screening for coeliac disease, since more specific blood tests are now available. These tests measure particular antibodies which are circulating in the blood. As was described earlier, antibodies are immunoglobulins which are made by the body's immune system against specific antigens. They indicate, therefore, that the body is mounting an immune reaction against something.

Anti-gliadin antibody (AGA) test

The first of these antibody tests in use in clinical practice was the one detecting antibodies against gliadin. It seems obvious that such a test should be developed for coeliac disease, since one would expect a coeliac patient to make antibodies against gliadin, the protein which is responsible for coeliac disease and which the body recognizes as an antigen.

Immunoglobulin type A (IgA) antibodies are normally measured since this is the main immunoglobulin involved in the gut immune response. In those people who are IgA deficient from birth, which we know is more common in coeliac disease, immunoglobulin type G (IgG) antibodies are produced by the body and these can be tested instead.

The important question with the antibody tests is how accurate are they? Estimates of accuracy are called the **sensitivity** and **specificity** of the test.

The average figures in Table 3 (page 68) reflect current medical experience. For IgA anti-gliadin antibodies (AGA-IgA), the average sensitivity is 78 per cent and the average specificity is 91 per cent. This means that of those people who truly have coeliac disease, the test will be positive in 78 per cent. This is its sensitivity, and means therefore that 22 per cent of people with coeliac disease could give a negative result (false negative). Hence the sensitivity is not good enough for a reliable screening test. The specificity is 91 per cent on average, which means that if coeliac disease is not present, the test is correct in 91 per cent of cases, with only nine per cent falsely positive. This means the test is quite specific since, if it is negative, it is likely that the individual does not have coeliac disease. However, this level of specificity, at an average of 91 per cent, is still not thought to be good enough for a reliable screening test.

The anti-endomysial antibody (EMA) test

In recent years more accurate tests have been developed. An antibody was discovered which was produced by the body against endomysium, which is a body tissue which supports and joins cells together. It was found that coeliac patients make antibodies against this tissue, the anti-endomysial antibodies (EMA-IgA). These have been tested for in many patients, like the AGA-IgA test. For EMA-IgA, the average sensitivity is 95 per cent and the average specificity is 99 per cent. These figures are much better than the AGA-IgA test, suggesting that the test detects 95 per cent

sensitivity
The measure of how well a diagnostic test detects a disease when it is present. For example, 90 per cent sensitivity means the test detects the disease in 9 out of 10 cases, but misses 1 in 10; that is a 'false negative' result. The closer the sensitivity gets to 100 per cent the more sensitive (i.e. better) the test is.

specificity
The measure of how often the result of a diagnostic test is negative when the disease is not present. For example, 90 per cent specificity means that in 9 out of 10 cases where the test is negative the patient does not have the disease, but in 1 in 10 the test is positive when, in fact, the disease is not present; a 'false positive' result. The closer the specificity gets to 100 per cent the more specific (i.e. better) the test is.

EMA
An antibody, usually made up of immunoglobulin A by the body, which reacts against an antigen called endomysium which is a body tissue. The antibody is made almost only by people who have coeliac disease.

of definite cases correctly, with five per cent falsely negative, and that it is so specific that only one per cent will be falsely positive. This latter figure means that if the test is negative, it is highly unlikely that the individual does have coeliac disease.

The tissue transglutaminase (tTG) test

Soon after the discovery of the EMA test, researchers found that the component of endomysium against which the antibody (EMA) was made was, in fact, an enzyme called **tissue transglutaminase (tTG)**. This enzyme is involved as the body repairs and remodels its tissues. This discovery made it much easier to develop a simpler test which measures tTG antibodies, and it was predicted that the results of this test would be very similar to the EMA-IgA test.

The average sensitivity is 90 per cent and the average specificity is 95 per cent. As can be seen, it is not quite as good as the EMA test; in definite cases it is correctly positive 90 per cent of the time, but ten per cent are falsely negative. Likewise, in 95 per cent of cases it accurately excludes coeliac disease, but in five per cent it is falsely positive.

In hospital laboratories, the tTG test is becoming routine, since it is a very simple and quick test to perform. If positive, it is usually checked with an EMA test. This means that most false positives can be reliably excluded. It does mean, however, that a few people will have a negative result when they do have coeliac disease.

These results highlight once again the need for careful interpretation of blood test results. If a

> **tissue transglutaminase (tTG)**
> An enzyme in the body which is part of the endomysium tissue. An antibody almost identical to EMA is made against tTG but is easier to detect in a laboratory test. This is an anti-tTG antibody.

doctor has a strong clinical suspicion of coeliac disease, despite a negative blood test, then a small intestinal biopsy would still be desirable.

A very small number of people who have a false positive result will go on to have a biopsy which will turn out to be normal. However, undergoing a biopsy is probably less of a problem than taking an unnecessary gluten-free diet for the long term. These findings confirm that the EMA and tTG tests are satisfactory for screening for coeliac disease, but should not be used as the definitive diagnostic test (Table 3).

Q **What should I do if I have a positive blood test suggesting coeliac disease?**

A You have presumably had the blood test because of symptoms which suggest coeliac disease may be present, or because you have been found to have a nutritional deficiency such as anaemia, or perhaps because you have a relative with coeliac disease. It is important that a diagnosis is properly made. In the present state of medical knowledge, it is recommended that a biopsy test is performed, while you are still taking a normal (gluten-containing) diet. You must resist the temptation to start a gluten-free diet since this can affect the biopsy test result and could cause the diagnosis to be questioned, particularly in the future if you continue to have symptoms, or develop any new ones.

An important final comment on the antibody tests is that they are believed to have very similar reliability and accuracy for children and adults alike, although they have been less extensively tested in children. Unfortunately, in children below the age of two, we do not have enough information to say how reliable they are. In the future it is to be expected that even more accurate blood tests will be developed which will probably obviate the need for biopsies in many cases.

Table 3 Average sensitivities and specificities for many published series of results in coeliac disease

IgA antibody tests	Sensitivity	Specificity
AGA	78%	91%
EMA	95%	99%
tTG	90%	95%

myth
Coeliac disease can definitely be diagnosed by a blood test.

fact
This is not true. The blood tests measure antibody levels and, although more than 90 per cent accurate, there is still the possibility of occasional false-positive or false-negative results. Blood tests are very helpful but should not be relied upon solely. In the future they may well become 100 per cent reliable.

The small intestinal biopsy

As already described in some detail, coeliac disease principally affects the small intestine, and the diagnosis is still most reliably made by obtaining a biopsy from this part of the intestine.

Many patients who were diagnosed years ago will have memories of swallowing the early biopsy capsules and waiting several hours for them to reach the correct place in the small intestine before a biopsy could be taken. Even then, the mechanism sometimes failed and no biopsy was obtained. Nowadays things have vastly improved and modern, flexible endoscopes are used. The endoscopist can watch on a television screen as the endoscope passes down the oesophagus, through the stomach and into the duodenum. The patient can choose to have

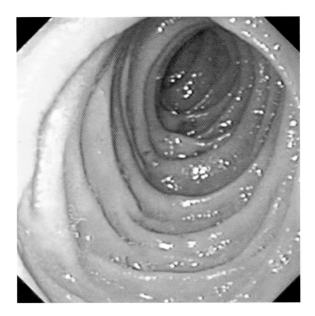

PLATE 1 A view of the inside of the small intestine using an endoscope.

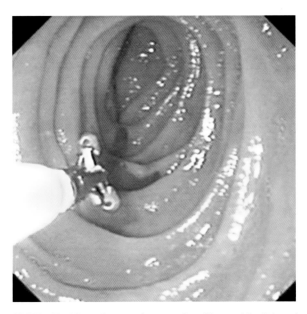

PLATE 2 The biopsy forceps about to take a biopsy of the lining of the small intestine.

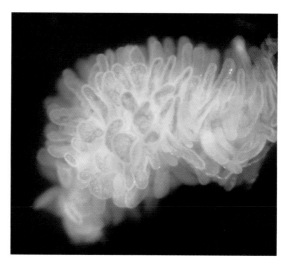

PLATE 3 A normal small intestinal biopsy showing villi (approximately 10 x normal size).

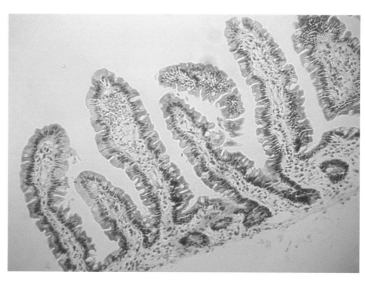

PLATE 4 A microscopic section of a normal small intestinal biopsy (approximately 40 x normal size).

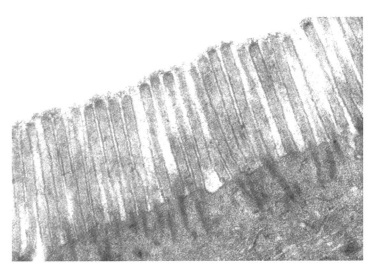

PLATE 5 Electron micrograph showing normal microvilli on the surface of an enterocyte (approximately 40,000 x normal size).

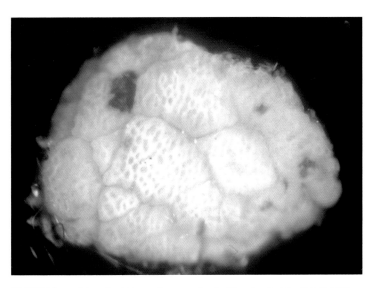

PLATE 6 A small intestinal biopsy from a patient with untreated coeliac disease (approximately 10 x normal size).

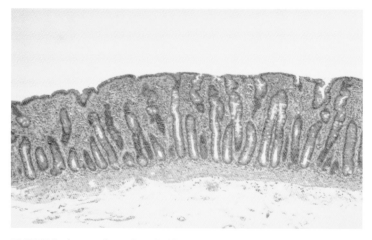

PLATE 7 A microscopic section of a biopsy from an untreated coeliac patient. There are no villi but deep crypts (approximately 40 x normal size).

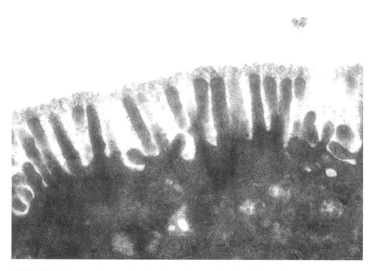

PLATE 8 Electron micrograph showing abnormal microvilli on the surface of an enterocyte from a patient with untreated coeliac disease.

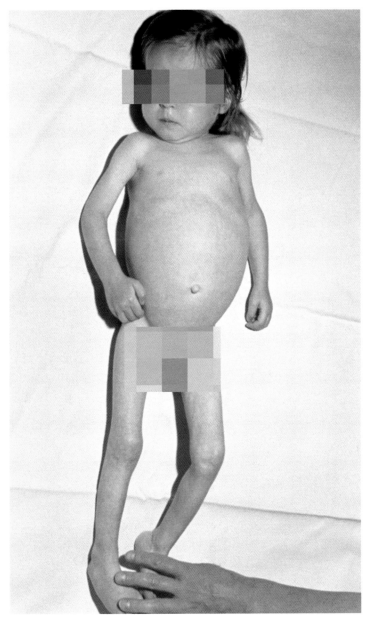

PLATE 9 A child diagnosed with coeliac disease at age two. The child is underweight with a swollen abdomen.

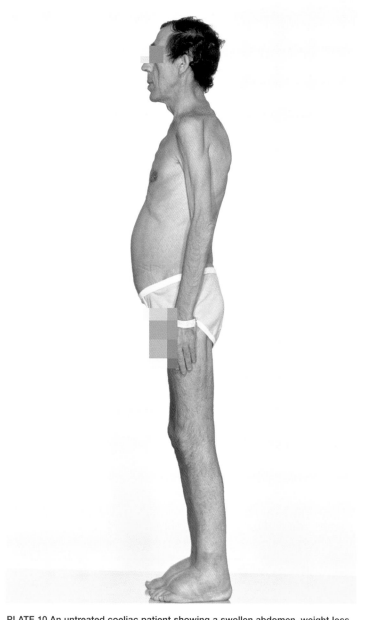

PLATE 10 An untreated coeliac patient showing a swollen abdomen, weight loss around the upper body and swollen ankles.

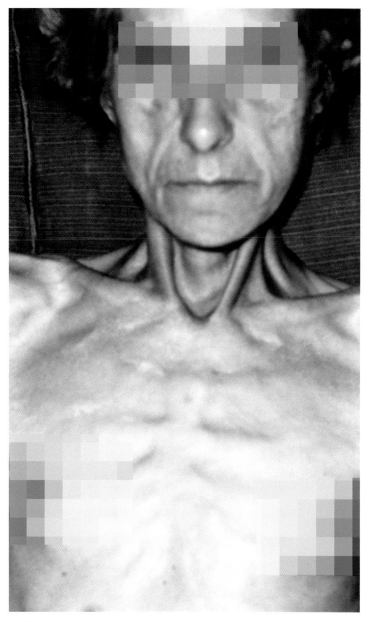

PLATE 11 An untreated patient with weakness, severe weight loss and diarrhoea.

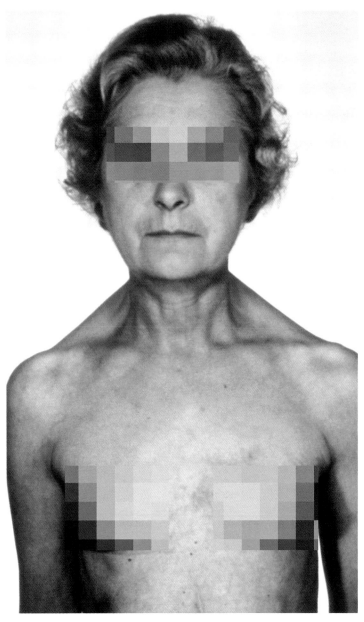

PLATE 12 The same patient as in Plate 11 after six months' treatment with a gluten-free diet.

mild sedation, or just a local anaesthetic spray to the back of the throat. It only takes a few minutes to reach the part of the duodenum where biopsies can be taken. This is shown in Plates 1 and 2. Having a biopsy taken does not cause any pain.

my experience

When I was first diagnosed with coeliac disease I had to have an endoscopy test to get a biopsy of the lining of the intestine. That was the thing I was dreading most. It sounded awful when I heard about it from a neighbour who had had one. She didn't have coeliac disease, but she had had a duodenal ulcer which had been bleeding.

However, it wasn't as bad as I expected, thank God! I received a letter from the hospital with a date and time. Fortunately there was a drop-off space outside the out-patient ward, so my son dropped me off there. He had been asked to come back at lunchtime to pick me up and to make sure that there was someone at home with me until the next day.

The nurse was very helpful when I went in. She took my personal and medical details, made sure I was on no medication and that I had had nothing to eat or drink since midnight. She also checked my pulse and blood pressure, but I didn't need to get undressed, only to make sure I had no tight clothes on.

I had already decided to have some sedation when the nurse asked me. Apparently half the patients choose to have a throat spray to numb the back of the throat, but are awake; the other half (which included me!) have an injection into a vein in the arm, which is a sedative like a quick-acting sleeping tablet. It is not an anaesthetic, but you certainly don't remember much of what happens. Of course, if you have the injection, you have to stay in the hospital for a few hours, but if you have the throat spray you can get up and go home straightaway.

The endoscopist, who was a specialist nurse, was very good. She quickly checked my details and explained what an endoscopy was and any risks, which are, in fact, very small indeed.

However, I was still afraid of the unknown! She then asked me if I was happy to sign the consent form, which had already been sent to me with the appointment letter. It is certainly quite detailed and legal, but the nurse explained what it meant. I was also asked if I minded the biopsies being used for medical research into coeliac disease. I certainly didn't mind that since it is important to know more about coeliac disease.

I then lay down on my left side on a hospital trolley and the nurse put a thin plastic tube into a vein in my arm – that was probably the worst part of the whole process! She then infused an injection, which felt cold as it went up my arm. I slowly felt a bit drunk then and far away. I could feel them putting something in my mouth and coughing, but it was all a bit vague and I don't remember much about it. In no time at all I was sitting up on the trolley in the next room, which was about 30 minutes later. It was all over.

I stayed until lunchtime and they checked my pulse and blood pressure regularly. I had some tea and then my son took me home. For the rest of the day I felt tired and my throat was sore, but otherwise I was fine. I had a good night's sleep after all the worry and was back to normal the next day.

My doctor says that I may need another biopsy some time, but I won't worry like I did last time. OK, it's not the best experience, but it's certainly not the worst!

Although the endoscopy is being performed to obtain biopsies, obviously the upper part of the gastrointestinal tract can be examined carefully at the same time for any other medical conditions. The whole examination will only take approximately ten to 15 minutes. This is all a significant improvement from the early days of biopsy tests. If it is necessary to take biopsies from children, this would usually be done under a short general anaesthetic.

The enteroscope

Endoscopes have been made which are longer than those in routine use and are called **enteroscopes**. These can be used to look further down, past the duodenum into the jejunum (the next part of the small intestine) (see Chapter 2). These are more difficult to use, and only specialist centres will have one. Biopsies can be obtained at different sites in the small intestine and such an instrument would be useful if it was thought a patient might have a complication of coeliac disease (see Chapter 6). Complications are very rare, however, and since the disease affects the upper small intestine more than the lower small intestine, adequate representative biopsies from the upper part, that is the duodenum, obtained using a normal endoscope, are satisfactory for almost all diagnostic purposes.

enteroscope
An endoscope which is longer than normal. It is made so that it can reach further down into the small intestine. It is more difficult to manipulate than the usual endoscope.

Video capsule endoscopy

Capsule endoscopies are now available. These involve swallowing a capsule (the size of a large lozenge) which contains a minute camera and radio transmitter. The capsule travels down the intestine, taking about eight hours on average before being passed and discarded when the bowels are opened. All the time the camera is taking pictures of the inside of the intestine and transmitting them to a recorder which the patient wears around his or her waist. There is thus a record of the appearance of the whole of the small intestinal mucosa. This will show any abnormalities. It can be used to look for complications of coeliac disease, but the capsule cannot take biopsies and is not used routinely for the diagnosis or follow-up of coeliac disease.

What the pathologist looks for

Once a biopsy is obtained, it is sent to the laboratory for processing. The tissue is preserved in a small block of paraffin wax and then very thin slivers are cut vertically through the block, each of which will contain a fine section of the biopsy. This is placed on a glass microscope slide and is stained with various dyes, which make the cells predominantly red and blue colours, so that the structure can be seen down a microscope. The paraffin block can be kept indefinitely so that at any time, even years later, slivers can be cut to review the biopsy and check on the diagnosis and progress if needed.

Examples of these slivers or histological sections are shown in Plates 4 and 7, showing a normal mucosal section and an untreated coeliac mucosal section respectively.

Making a definite diagnosis of coeliac disease

As we have seen, coeliac disease is a disease in which there is an abnormality affecting the small intestine in genetically predisposed individuals, precipitated by the ingestion of gluten-containing foods. It is in this definition that the criteria for making a definite diagnosis can be found.

Clearly, it suggests:

✧ that the small intestine should be examined
✧ that there may be a recognizable genetic make-up of patients

◇ that they would have gluten-containing food in their diet.

In the present state of knowledge, we are not able to perform a definite diagnostic genetic test. However, we can obtain a piece of small intestine in a biopsy and we do know what type of diet patients are taking. In most patients, making the diagnosis is straightforward and we are helped by having available the antibody blood tests to support the diagnosis.

The diagnostic pathway

Obviously, coeliac disease has to be thought of in the first place, and the clinical suspicion raised. This may be because of the classical symptoms, atypical features or associated conditions, as described in Chapter 4. The diagnostic pathway shown in Figure 5.1 is then a logical way forward.

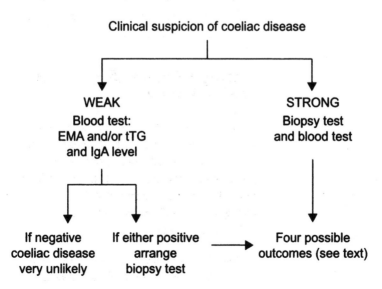

Figure 5.1 The diagnostic pathway for coeliac diease.

As can be seen, if the clinical suspicion is weak and an antibody blood test is negative, it is very unlikely that the patient has coeliac disease. If, however, symptoms persist, or develop, a further blood test may be worthwhile, and even a biopsy test may be indicated. A positive blood test should lead on to a biopsy test. If the clinical suspicion is strong, after ensuring the patient is on a gluten-containing diet, one should proceed to both antibody blood test and a biopsy test. This can lead to four outcomes:

1 Antibody and biopsy positive – coeliac disease confirmed.
2 Antibody positive and biopsy negative – keep patient under review, potential coeliac disease, consider repeat biopsy later.
3 Antibody negative and biopsy positive – consider other rare cause of mucosal abnormality but otherwise treat as coeliac disease, possible false negative antibody result.
4 Antibody and biopsy negative – coeliac disease excluded.

Remaining questions

By following the above diagnostic pathway, the clinical situation becomes clear for the vast majority of patients seeking a definite diagnosis. There are some remaining questions which arise.

A second biopsy

For many years, once a patient had started a gluten-free diet, it was recommended that a second biopsy should be obtained after six to 12 months of the diet, to make sure the mucosa was returning to normal. Nowadays, if the patient is improving clinically while taking a gluten-free diet, and the positive antibody test becomes negative, then a second biopsy is not absolutely necessary. Some doctors however, and also some patients, do like to check for mucosal improvement with a biopsy test. Follow-up biopsies in other circumstances are discussed in Chapter 6.

Q **Now that I have been taking a gluten-free diet for 12 months and feel very well, how often do I need biopsy tests of my intestine?**

A As you know, a biopsy obtained at the time of an endoscopy test is necessary to make the diagnosis of coeliac disease confidently (see Chapter 5). If the patient then improves and the clinical problems resolve, then a follow-up biopsy is not mandatory; however, some coeliac specialists and also patients like to confirm the improvement with a further biopsy which should show healing of the intestine. If there is any doubt about the diagnosis or remaining clinical problems, a follow-up biopsy is required. Patients should be under long-term follow-up either by the hospital specialist or the GP and, over the years, a repeat biopsy may be recommended, particularly if there is a return of symptoms or a query arises about the diagnosis or a possible complication. Some patients are strongly reassured if they have a biopsy test every few years which shows continued normality of the intestine.

The need for follow-up biopsies in children has caused more discussion over the years. This is because in children under the age of two years, a biopsy can be abnormal due to other food intolerances as well as gluten. The antibody tests are also not as helpful, since at this age there is relatively little information about their reliability.

Thus, in many children, once a gluten-free diet has been taken for between one and two years, many paediatricians would be reassured to see a biopsy result which shows improvement from the initial one. At one time, in the 1970s and 1980s, paediatricians even required a **gluten 'challenge'** with gluten being re-introduced in order to provoke a mucosal abnormality in order to confirm the diagnosis. This is now no longer considered appropriate. In rare cases, in which children have been given gluten-free diets without biopsy evidence, the diagnosis can be difficult, and a gluten 'challenge' may have to be considered. It may also have to be considered when older children question the need for life-long gluten restriction, particularly if the initial diagnosis has not been adequately confirmed.

gluten challenge
The deliberate ingestion of food containing a known amount of gluten in order to produce the symptoms or small intestinal mucosal abnormalities suggestive of coeliac disease. It is used when there is doubt about the definite diagnosis of coeliac disease.

Q My daughter was diagnosed with coeliac disease at 12 months of age by a biopsy test, which showed the typical features of coeliac disease. She is now 12 years old and very well on a gluten-free diet. Does she need a gluten challenge?

A No, she does not need a gluten challenge. She is probably at the time of the adolescent growth spurt and it is important she develops normally; a gluten challenge could affect this. If as a young adult she questions the diagnosis of coeliac disease, further biopsies could be obtained in relation to altering the gluten in her diet. It is better to leave well alone at present.

Other causes of mucosal disease

In outcome 3 above (page 74), reference was made to other rare causes of an abnormal biopsy. In developed countries these are very rare, but may have to be considered by the specialist if

Table 4 Conditions with an abnormal small intestinal mucosa which may resemble coeliac disease

Infections: giardia, tuberculosis, HIV, gastroenteritis in children
Tropical sprue
Food intolerance: cow's milk, or soya protein intolerance in children
Immunodeficiency states
Eosinophilic gastroenteritis
Small bowel bacterial overgrowth syndrome
Whipple's disease
Crohn's disease
Arterial disease
Drug and radiation damage
Zollinger-Ellison syndrome
Severe malnutrition

there is any doubt. A list for such consideration is given in Table 4. A description of these disorders is beyond the scope of this book.

The extent of the abnormality in the small intestinal mucosa

Although coeliac disease affects the small intestinal mucosa, there is considerable variation between patients as to its extent. In all patients, the duodenal mucosa will be involved, but how far down it extends varies from one person to another. In most it will not be extensive, thus leaving enough normal mucosa lower down to maintain absorption of nutrients sufficient to keep the body functioning even if not entirely normally. The extent of the abnormality probably correlates with the severity of the gastrointestinal symptoms. There is no easy way to measure the extent of the disease.

myth
The whole of the intestine is abnormal in coeliac disease.

fact
The main abnormalities found in coeliac disease occur in the mucosa of the small intestine, and they are worse in the first few feet. Any abnormalities that occur further down in the small intestine are much milder and these quickly improve with treatment. Detailed examination of biopsies from the stomach or the colon of the coeliac patient can show increased numbers of lymphocytes related to the underlying immune reaction in coeliac disease. These, however, do not cause medical problems for the patient.

The severity of the abnormality in the small intestinal mucosa

In outcomes 1 and 3 above (page 74), a positive biopsy test was mentioned. This implies definite features of the typical coeliac abnormality, described in Chapter 2, that is reduced height of the villi, increased depth of the crypts and increased numbers of immune cells (mainly lymphocytes). The severity of these abnormalities can also vary between patients and even, to a small extent, between biopsies from one patient. Hence, the biopsies should always be examined by a pathologist with experience of coeliac mucosal abnormalities.

Specialists in coeliac disease now classify the degree of abnormality into grades (0–4). This grading system was originally developed by Dr Michael Marsh, a physician who worked for many years in Manchester.

Grade 0 Normal mucosa, but positive antibody tests ('pre-infiltrative').

Grade 1 Increased infiltration by lymphocytes in the epithelium, but normal villi and crypts ('infiltrative').

Grade 2 Increased infiltration by lymphocytes, increased depth of crypts, normal villous length ('infiltrative and hyperplastic').

Grade 3 Increased infiltration by lymphocytes, deep crypts, reduced villous height ('flat, destructive', classical features of untreated coeliac disease).

Grade 4 Loss of villi, reduced crypts, fewer lymphocytes ('atrophic, hypoplastic', severe complicated coeliac disease very rare).

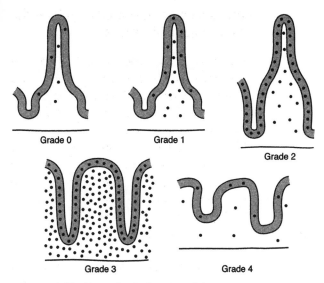

Figure 5.2 Marsh's grading for the mucosal changes seen in coeliac disease. Grades 2 and 3 are the most common changes seen at diagnosis. These include reduced or absent villi, increased depth to the crypts and increased number of lymphocytes. On treatment with a gluten-free diet, the mucosa improves back towards Grade 0.

These grades are shown diagrammatically in Figure 5.2.

Individuals with Grade 0 are those in outcome 2 above; they are the potential coeliacs in the coeliac iceberg (Chapter 3) and should be kept under medical review. Those with Grades 1–4 will have had positive antibody tests at some stage. Grade 1 patients will most probably have no symptoms. Those patients with Grade 2 and 3 abnormalities are the most common, including the vast majority of coeliac patients. Those with the severe Grade 4 abnormality are very rare and have a serious medical condition, discussed in Chapter 6.

Why there is a variation in severity is unknown, but it probably reflects biological variation, the genetic inheritance of the individual patient and environmental factors, particularly the amount of gluten taken at various stages during their lives.

Further tests

When a patient seeks medical help and has gastrointestinal symptoms in particular, diagnoses other than coeliac disease have to be considered, and often other investigations are performed.

CT scan

A CT (computerized tomography) scan is a series of detailed X-rays taken by a scanning machine, which are then put together by a computer to give detailed pictures of the part of the body which is scanned.

A **CT scan** or ultrasound scan of the abdomen may be arranged. These may show some swelling or increased fluid in the intestine, and some slightly enlarged lymph nodes for example. Such findings, while being compatible with coeliac disease, do not confirm the diagnosis. However, they may suggest the need for a biopsy test.

Similarly, a barium X-ray may be arranged. Barium in the stomach and small intestine may show an unusual pattern of dispersal suggestive of a small intestinal abnormality, once again indicating the need for a biopsy.

Several years ago, tests of how various substances were absorbed from the small intestine were used, but these were not specific for coeliac disease, only perhaps suggesting that there was a disease there. Nowadays, the increased ease of obtaining endoscopic biopsies, and the increased accuracy of antibody blood tests, has made such tests unnecessary in diagnosis.

myth

Many people must have coeliac disease, since they are better on a wheat-free or gluten-free diet.

fact

Food intolerance is said to be very common and many people omit various foods from their diet and find that their gastrointestinal symptoms improve. This includes some people who find they feel better by omitting wheat or gluten-containing products. The author has seen many such people. In many there is no doubt they are intolerant to the particular food, but they do not have coeliac disease. Coeliac disease is a very characteristic disease with biopsy abnormalities specifically related to gluten in the diet. People with food intolerance have normal biopsies and negative coeliac blood tests while taking wheat or gluten in their diet. The medical basis for food intolerances is unknown at present.

CHAPTER

6

Looking after a patient with coeliac disease

Once coeliac disease has been properly diagnosed, treatment can begin. It is apparent from the variety of symptoms which patients have that treatment may have to be tailored to their individual needs. The cornerstone of treatment is, of course, life-long adherence to a gluten-free diet. Other treatment, however, may be necessary in patients who have severe symptoms initially. For example, patients may be found to be seriously deficient in vitamins, minerals and blood. They will require intravenous replacement, including blood transfusion, and even intravenous feeding. This used to be more common many years ago, but nowadays would be extremely rare.

It is much more likely that the treatment recommended will be a gluten-free diet for life, together with some vitamin supplements for a few months to replenish any deficiency, for example iron and/or folic acid tablets.

The gluten-free diet

Recommending and starting a gluten-free diet (**GFD**) is a major step and has widespread implications for the patient and his or her family and friends. In many areas of the world, including Europe, North and South America, Australasia and North Africa, gluten-containing cereals form part of the staple diet. Gluten-rich products such as bread and pasta are basic to the normal diet; they make a substantial contribution to the daily energy intake and are palatable and easy to eat. Changing to a GFD and maintaining it as a life-long treatment is a major step and has a substantial impact on daily life. This has to be handled well and sympathetically by medical, nursing and dietetic staff. The role of an experienced dietitian is invaluable for the coeliac patient.

> **GFD (gluten-free diet)**
> The diet to treat people with coeliac disease. To be free of gluten, the food eaten must not contain wheat, barley, rye or their products.

Where is gluten found?

As we saw in Chapter 3, gluten is derived from wheat, rye and barley. A GFD therefore consists of excluding foods containing products of these three cereals.

What about oats?

There has been a lot of discussion about oats, since this is a related cereal, but the gluten equivalent in oats is now thought to be safe to eat by the vast majority of coeliac patients. There are some good studies in coeliac patients showing that neither their symptoms nor biopsies deteriorate if they eat oats as part of a GFD. There is a problem in day-to-day life, however, since sometimes manufacturers will use the same mill to grind oats as wheat or barley. This can lead to contamination of oats. Hence, patients should, if at all possible, use pure oats or products made by specialist manufacturers who can guarantee purity. Some coeliac specialists believe that there may be a very small number of coeliac patients who are truly sensitive to the gluten fraction in oats, but these, if they exist, must be very rare.

What about wheat starch?

As described in Chapter 3, the gluten proteins can be removed from wheat flour, leaving **wheat starch**, which is a rich source of carbohydrate. There is always the chance that all the gluten cannot be removed, leaving a trace amount in the starch. However, for the last 50 years wheat starch has been allowed in the United Kingdom as part of a GFD. This is specially prepared wheat starch which can be included in labelled gluten-free foods. (It is called **Codex wheat starch** since it is specially defined by international agreement to a specific standard, or code.) In some European countries, in Australia and in North America, even this wheat starch is not allowed. However, many studies have shown that there is no difference in the symptoms or biopsies of coeliac patients who take a GFD which does or does not contain this wheat starch. The very low level of gluten in such wheat starch does not affect the small intestinal mucosa of the vast majority of patients. However, occasionally a patient does not fully return to normal and omitting food which contains wheat starch does help. These patients, in fact, are then taking a gluten-free, wheat-free diet.

wheat starch
The principal constituent of flour, which is produced by milling wheat seeds.

Codex wheat starch
Wheat starch which, after milling, is only permitted to have a very small amount of gluten remaining, as laid down by an international standard, and is therefore able to be eaten by most coeliac patients.

What is allowed?

It must be stressed that a GFD can be very palatable and nutritious. Natural foods, such as vegetables, salads, pulses, fruits, nuts, meat, fish, poultry, cheese, eggs and milk can all be eaten. Historically, rice, maize (corn) and potatoes were the substitutes for the gluten-containing cereals. A number of grains, seeds, legumes and nut flours are now available, which offer more variety, improved palatability and higher nutritional quality to a GFD. These are shown in Table 5.

Dietary advice

In implementing the GFD, the coeliac patient needs a lot of support, hence the need for an experienced dietitian. So often in the past

myth
A gluten-free diet is unhealthy.

fact
A gluten-free diet can be very healthy. Patients usually take more meat, fish, fruit and vegetables than normal, and of course have to eliminate snack foods made with gluten-containing flour such as biscuits and cakes or pastries. Patients can obtain adequate carbohydrate from gluten-free alternatives, which may include rice, corn and potatoes as well as special gluten-free bread and pasta products.

myth
Corn (maize) is a type of wheat.

fact
Corn is often used as an overall term for any cereal crop. However, it is more accurately a word used as an alternative name for maize. Although this is a food crop, it is not at all closely related to wheat and does not contain gluten.

Table 5 Grains, seeds and other starch sources

Allowed in a GFD	Not allowed in a GFD
Amaranth	Wheat (includes spelt, semolina,
Arrowroot	durum)
Buckwheat	Rye
Corn/maize	Barley
Indian rice grass	
Legumes	
Mesquite	
Millet	
Nuts	
Potato	
Quinoa	
Rice	
Sorghum	
Soy	
Tapioca	
Teff	
Wild rice	
Oats	see text
Codex wheat starch	

outdated or incorrect information was produced and no further help offered. Many patients require time to learn about nutrition and the diet in particular. This will be affected by their individual circumstances, their social situation, and their particular worries and anxieties. Some of these issues are mentioned in Chapter 7.

The dietitian will advise about cereals and such questions as those surrounding oats and Codex wheat starch referred to previously. They will also advise about the gluten content of processed foods. Many ready-made meals and convenience foods contain wheat-derived ingredients often added as coating, fillers or stabilizing agents. These include sausages, fish fingers, many soups and sauces, and some medications and vitamin preparations that you can buy over the counter. Barley is used in the manufacture of many alcoholic drinks but ales, beers, stouts and lagers are the only ones that should be avoided. Recently some gluten-free beers have been manufactured. Spirits, wines, liqueurs, sherry, port and cider are allowed. Whisky and malt whisky are allowed as distilled spirits are gluten-free irrespective of the cereal used in the production.

Malt extract and malt flavouring are both manufactured from barley and widely used in the food industry. The quantity of barley-derived ingredient used in products varies. Products that contain malt extract in smaller amounts can usually be tolerated by most people with coeliac disease, for example, malt vinegar, but some malted breakfast cereals have been shown to have a higher level of gluten than previously realized and these products may not be so suitable in a gluten-free diet.

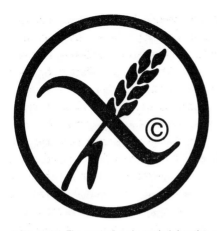

Figure 6.1 The crossed-grain symbol denoting a gluten-free product, registered by Coeliac UK.

Developments in gluten testing, with improvements in accuracy, are helping us to understand more about the safe limits for people on a gluten-free diet. It is because of these developments that regular dietetic advice is helpful, and also why patients should be given information about their national Coeliac Society (Coeliac UK in the United Kingdom). Such societies publish information on the gluten-free diet and coeliac disease and regularly update gluten-free food lists. They have on-going contact with food manufacturers and exchange information on the ingredients in foods available in supermarkets, health-food stores and on prescription. They are influential in persuading manufacturers and suppliers to increase their ranges of gluten-free products and in improving labelling. Many supermarket chains have greatly increased their range of gluten-free products in recent years. The crossed-grain symbol, registered by Coeliac UK, for gluten-free products is well known (see Figure 6.1).

In the UK, new regulations for food labelling which help to identify foods that contain gluten have been introduced. These are more informative and make it necessary for the manufacturer to list all ingredients nowadays. There is one unfortunate issue, however. Some products, which have not actually changed, will now have to be labelled as containing gluten or as wheat products, since they have always had a very low level of gluten, (only just detectable), which is not detrimental to the vast majority of coeliac patients. This will inevitably lead to some confusion. If in doubt, always check with the manufacturer, retailer, a dietitian or Coeliac UK.

Response to treatment

The great majority of patients begin to feel better within weeks of starting a GFD. In young children their appetite and mood changes within days and they begin to grow properly, reaching their predicted height and weight within months. Most adults also respond well, and within a few weeks or months are feeling healthy (see Plates 11 and 12). It is more difficult to predict an improvement in people who have had virtually no symptoms, perhaps having been discovered by family screening, or because they have mild anaemia. However, even these patients often say that they feel generally more healthy and that they never realized previously they had been under par.

Q **Once on a gluten-free diet, what will happen?**

A Initially you will presumably find it rather strange and somewhat difficult to stick to the diet. Gluten will be found to be in some processed foods you never imagined it would be! If you have had symptoms of diarrhoea or stomach pains or tiredness, these should begin to improve within two to three weeks, although the healing and continuing improvement will go on for many months. If you had virtually no symptoms, then you may not feel any different, although it is likely that you will find you have more energy.

Q **What other treatment may be necessary in addition to a gluten-free diet?**

A In the vast majority of coeliac patients, the only other treatment necessary is some vitamin and mineral supplements. These may include iron,

A calcium, multi-vitamins, folic acid and Vitamin D. They are often used initially to top up your levels, but eventually patients will obtain all they need from their diet once they are well treated. Long-term use of recommended doses is safe, however. Such use should be discussed on an individual basis with your doctor or dietitian.

Some potential problems

Despite a good response to treatment, however, there are some potential problems. Most patients put on weight once treatment is started. Obviously this is welcome in many cases, and reflects the improving intestinal mucosa with increased absorption of nutrients. However, some patients will become overweight. This will be due to a combination of factors: they feel better and have an increased appetite, and there is increased absorption in the intestine. In such cases, dietary advice about weight management may be necessary.

Conversely, some patients find the GFD difficult to manage and become frightened to eat anything other than very obviously gluten-free foods. Hence, their overall intake is insufficient and they lose weight. Obviously, they need strong and sympathetic dietary support.

It will be obvious that if patients are avoiding cereals such as wheat, barley and rye, their diet could potentially lack normal sources of **fibre** (for example, the husks or bran from these cereal grains). This reduced intake of fibre can lead to quite severe constipation, especially if patients have that tendency anyway. Plenty of fruit, vegetables and pulses are therefore recom-mended. Brown rice and wholemeal or granary gluten-free bread and wholemeal gluten-free pasta

fibre
The indigestible constituent of plant foods, which forms 'roughage' or bulk to the intestinal contents, and hence helps to keep the intestinal peristalsis functioning and bowels opening normally.

are also recommended to increase fibre intake. Gluten-free muesli made from brown rice and millet with added seeds, nuts and dried fruits is a great way to start the day and provides a high-fibre breakfast cereal. Otherwise, if tolerated, pure oats provides a high-fibre cereal on the gluten-free diet. If necessary, rice or soya bran is available, as well as ispaghula husk or methyl cellulose. These are all safe and provide bulk to the intestinal contents, thus helping to relieve constipation.

Compliance with a GFD

Taking a GFD is a major change in a person's life, and there are bound to be difficulties. Some patients find it easier than others to comply with the diet, which will partly reflect their underlying personality, self-discipline or laid-back attitude to life in general. Many surveys of patients have been performed to look at compliance with a GFD; these show that between 45 per cent and 95 per cent of patients adhere to a strict diet. Such surveys depend, of course, on the population of patients surveyed, and may partly reflect the availability of local medical and dietary support.

There is a number of specific reasons why people find it difficult to stick to a GFD:

✧ The diet imposes some restrictions on everyday lifestyle.
✧ It is more difficult to eat out while travelling, on holiday or meeting friends.
✧ Young children find birthday and other parties difficult.
✧ Adolescents find 'being different' very difficult, and bow to peer pressure to conform and eat acceptable teenage food.

- ✧ Adolescents frequently get few symptoms from eating gluten-containing foods and therefore think it is all right to do so.
- ✧ Patients with 'silent' coeliac disease also get few symptoms, if any, while taking gluten in their diet, so there is little incentive to stick to a strict diet.
- ✧ A GFD is probably more expensive than a normal diet.

Is there a risk to consuming a small amount of gluten?

Ideally, doctors recommend that a GFD should be always as strict as possible. However, as we have learnt in this chapter, a totally gluten-free diet may be very difficult to achieve for a variety of reasons.

There is some evidence in studies in coeliac patients that very small amounts of gluten have no significant effects on the small intestinal mucosa. Hence, there does appear to be a very low level which may be safe. This is why specially manufactured wheat starch, which could have a low level of gluten contamination, is used safely in the UK in many gluten-free products. Supporting evidence for this safety comes from the fact that many studies showing the benefits of gluten withdrawal from the diet, including reducing the risk of complications, have employed a GFD which allows wheat starch. Not surprisingly, there is a very small number of patients who are incredibly sensitive to even traces of gluten, and these people will often need to take a very strict wheat-free, gluten-free diet. Such patients even avoid normal communion wafers to which they find themselves sensitive and need to check all medication with the pharmacist, since often wheat

myth
Taking gluten by mistake is dangerous.

fact
Usually when we think about 'dangerous' medical conditions we imagine they are life-threatening. Inadvertent consumption of gluten is not that dangerous. In fact, some patients have no effects they are aware of. Others, however, can develop quite marked gastrointestinal effects within a few hours. All gluten has some effects on the small intestinal mucosa in coeliac patients, whether or not symptoms occur. Hence it is better to try to stick to a strict gluten-free diet. However, you should not be frightened if you find you have made a mistake and eaten something containing gluten.

flour is used as a 'filler' (non-active ingredient) in tablets or capsules.

Q **Can I stray off my gluten-free diet occasionally? What harm will it do to me?**

A The correct theoretical answer is no, you should not stray from your gluten-free diet. However, practically, for some people this may be very difficult. Some patients are very sensitive to even a small amount of gluten and would immediately get symptoms. This is a strong incentive to stay on the diet. Others get no symptoms if they take gluten-containing food. Any gluten will produce some change to the intestinal lining, whether or not it gives symptoms. The more gluten, the more abnormalities will be induced. Taking a small amount of gluten on very infrequent occasions should allow the intestine to heal in between times; regular gluten will lead to continual abnormalities. A continually abnormal intestine, whether there are symptoms or not, can lead to complications such as recurrent anaemia, worsening osteoporosis or, rarely, gastrointestinal malignancy. The best advice is therefore to stick to the diet as strictly as possible, but do not panic if you make an occasional mistake with it.

Prognosis of coeliac disease

The prognosis, that is the expected outcome of the disease on treatment, in coeliac disease is excellent. At least 90 per cent of patients return to normal health and lead normal lives. There are treated coeliac patients who are Olympic athletes or who have climbed Mount Everest.

Obviously there are many symptoms which can occur in untreated patients, which eventually lead to the diagnosis being made, as described in Chapter 4. These would be expected to improve on treatment, as the disease improved. There are some associated conditions, also outlined in

Chapter 4, and these would be treated on their own merits, irrespective of coeliac disease. Hence some patients may have ongoing medical problems in such cases.

Well-treated patients have a normal life expectancy. In studies of untreated patients there is a slightly increased risk of earlier death due to the small number of patients who develop a very rare intestinal malignancy, but this risk is eliminated with good treatment of coeliac disease. This complication is discussed later in this chapter.

> **Q** **I have had coeliac disease for several years now and am taking a gluten-free diet. Is it safe to travel, or might it make my symptoms worse?**
>
> **A** In general it is safe for people with coeliac disease to travel. The usual precautions for anyone travelling should be taken but, there are extra problems for coeliac patients. Clearly, the gluten-free diet is more difficult in some places than others. European countries are similar to the UK in general, as is North America and Australia (see Chapter 7). Coeliac patients, especially if only relatively well-treated, may be more prone to the effects of gastroenteritis, so care with clean water and food preparation is important.

Patients who do not respond to treatment

There is a small number of patients who do not improve, or at least not fully, on treatment with a gluten-free diet. Most of these will have remaining symptoms but, in a few, it will be the biopsy abnormalities which are shown not to improve when follow-up biopsies have been arranged.

There are several reasons why patients do not respond to treatment as expected and these include the following:

✧ continuing gluten ingestion
✧ incorrect initial diagnosis
✧ lactose intolerance
✧ other food intolerances
✧ inadequate pancreatic function
✧ microscopic colitis
✧ co-existent irritable bowel syndrome
✧ complications of coeliac disease

The first of these reasons is the continued ingestion of gluten, either inadvertently or knowingly. This is another reason why careful dietary follow-up is so often needed. Patients may think they are taking a strictly GFD, but it needs some informed detective work to discover a hidden source of gluten. Continued ingestion of gluten is, by far, the most common reason why patients do not improve or remain symptomatic. Regular follow-up with an experienced dietitian builds confidence from both sides and patients should not feel criticized in this situation. It is far better to try to understand what is going on and why, or whether gluten is being ingested, than to be overly critical or judgemental.

The second reason why patients may not be responding as expected is because the wrong diagnosis has been made, and they do not have coeliac disease. In Chapter 5, Table 4 lists other causes of an abnormal biopsy which should be considered by the medical specialist in this type of situation. A recent survey in England showed that ten per cent of cases which did not respond to a GFD were wrongly diagnosed and did not have coeliac disease. This figure is probably not typical, since the report was from a highly specialized unit which would, naturally, have many more unusual cases than a the usual hospital clinic or health centre.

Other reasons why patients remain symptomatic include **lactose** intolerance, which may occur independently of coeliac disease and requires a lactose-free diet in addition, at least for a time. Occasionally other food intolerances have been found in addition to coeliac disease, for example cow's milk protein, soya protein, chicken, tuna and eggs. It should be stressed that these intolerances are very rare and coeliac patients should not expect to have them. Inadequate pancreatic secretion of digestive enzymes may occur in longstanding untreated coeliac disease, and require replacement with enzyme-containing capsules, at least initially, before all symptoms resolve. Also associated with coeliac disease is a mild form of **colitis**, microscopic colitis, which causes diarrhoea and is only diagnosed on a biopsy of the colon, the large intestine. Although rare, this can cause continuing symptoms and requires specific medication with drugs for colitis. Irritable bowel syndrome is very common in the general population. It causes a disturbed bowel habit and abdominal pain or discomfort. It can, of course, occur coincidentally in people with coeliac disease and may in itself be a cause of continuing gastrointestinal problems.

Finally, there are some serious complications of coeliac disease which may cause a poor response to treatment, or a relapse in symptoms after initial improvement over months or years. These are extremely rare, and will be discussed at the end of this chapter.

lactose
The type of sugar contained in milk and dairy products.

colitis
An inflammation of the large intestine (the colon). Symptoms produced include diarrhoea, which may contain blood.

Follow-up of coeliac patients

Patients with coeliac disease should receive regular follow-up. This can be by a specialist in gastroenterology at a hospital clinic, by a general practitioner who has a particular interest in coeliac disease or by an experienced dietitian who has easy access to medical advice. A team approach ensures that up-to-date information and education in dietary matters can be provided for the patient and that the best possible care is given. Unfortunately, such follow-up is often not available or not arranged. This may be because, until several years ago, many doctors thought that once a patient had been started on a GFD they would remain well and not require regular review. Some patients also find it onerous to attend a clinic or health centre on a regular basis, and only wish for medical help if required.

A number of professional medical associations have produced guidelines for the follow-up of coeliac patients. These include the British Society of Gastroenterology, the Primary Care Society for Gastroenterology, the American Gastroenterological Association and the National Institutes of Health (US).

It must be remembered that guidelines for the care of any medical condition are only guidelines, and not mandatory regulations. However, they attempt to be the recommended best practice at the time and to be based on the most up-to-date medical evidence. They must be interpreted on an individual patient basis but provide general principles of clinical management for the best care of the patient.

A summary of the guidelines suggests the following:

1 The diagnosis of coeliac disease must include an initial biopsy and preferably a positive antibody blood test.
2 A life-long gluten-free diet should be recommended.
3 Initial follow-up should ensure response to the diet.
4 Regular follow-up at least annually thereafter should be arranged in order to see a doctor and a dietitian with experience in coeliac disease.
5 At follow-up
   - current symptoms, physical well-being and weight should be checked
   - dietary compliance should be discussed
   - routine blood tests should be checked (e.g. blood count, calcium, iron, folic acid, albumin levels, antibody test)
   - a bone scan should be considered
   - a need for further biopsy test should be considered
   - a possible need for special vaccination should be discussed (see below).
6 Coincident disease and complications should be sought.
7 Up-to-date information should be provided and membership of Coeliac UK (or other national coeliac society) discussed.

There are a number of points requiring further comment in these guidelines. The need for a further biopsy test is raised. This has already been discussed in Chapter 5 but, to reiterate, a follow-up biopsy several months after the diagnostic biopsy is not mandatory if the diagnostic biopsy was typical of coeliac disease, if the antibody blood test was positive and if symptoms have improved and the antibody test has become negative with a GFD. However, if there is doubt about any of these factors, a second biopsy is strongly recommended, particularly if the patient still has symptoms or they return.

Consideration of a bone scan is mentioned in the guidelines. 'Thinning' (i.e. reduced density and hence weakness) of the bones occurs as we all get older. This is more common and more severe in coeliac patients and hence the density of the bones should be measured. It is commonly suggested that adult patients should have a bone scan for bone mineral density (called dual energy X-ray absorptiometry, or a DEXA scan). They should have this at diagnosis, and in men after 55 years, and in women after the menopause. If the scan reveals reduced bone density, then treatment should be considered (see below when complications are discussed).

One final point under guidelines relates to the need for vaccination. Obviously routine vaccinations for all of us should be carried out as normal in childhood, adulthood and before foreign travel. However, there is a degree of malfunction of the spleen described in coeliac disease; this produces a slightly increased risk of **pneumococcal infections** (a common cause of pneumonia). In practice, this increased risk is not measurable, since we are all (with or without coeliac disease) exposed to so many infections in the community. Some medical practitioners recommend pneumococcal vaccination, however, as an extra safeguard. This may be wise in older patients who are debilitated due to other diseases, but it is not recommended routinely for coeliac patients and there is no good evidence of an excess of pneumonia cases in the coeliac

pneumococcal infection
This is an infection, usually pneumonia, caused by a particular bacterium (or bug) called streptococcus pneumoniae (or pneumococcus). It can usually be adequately treated with penicillin. However, severe infection can occur and can be dangerous and other antibiotics may have to be used. Young children and elderly people are more prone to this infection.

population. This should be discussed with a patient's doctor if there is any concern.

A useful summary for follow-up of coeliac disease was produced by the National Institutes of Health in the United States in 2005. This has six key elements in follow-up, based on the American spelling of 'celiac':

C consultation with a skilled dietitian

E education about the disease

L life-long adherence to a gluten-free diet

I identification and treatment of nutritional deficiencies

A access to an advocacy group (for example, Coeliac UK)

C continuous long-term follow-up by a multi-disciplinary team.

Complications of coeliac disease

When discussing the complications of coeliac disease, it is necessary to clarify what is meant. In Chapter 4 the clinical features of coeliac disease were described and, since these are so wide and varied, some conditions were included which might also be considered 'complications'. Many of these conditions can be found in association with coeliac disease, such as diabetes or thyroid disease, and are listed in Table 2 in Chapter 4. Other conditions are not typical for coeliac patients, even though they may produce the clinical features which lead to the diagnosis; these include unusual neurological (i.e. affecting the brain and/or nervous system) features and reduced fertility, which are discussed in Chapter 4 (see Table 1). Dermatitis herpetiformis is also discussed in Chapter 4. Many of these clinical features do improve on treatment of the coeliac disease with a GFD and the incidence of complications is also much reduced if a strict GFD is taken.

There are some specific complications which it is important to discuss in some detail.

Bone disease

The increased publicity about osteoporosis has brought bone disease to the fore when considering possible complications and follow-up of patients with coeliac disease. There are a number of reasons why coeliac patients may develop bone problems. Their intake of calcium may be reduced; the small intestinal abnormality will result in decreased absorption into the body of both calcium and **Vitamin D** and the coeliac abnormality may result in even more calcium being lost from the body. The metabolism of calcium, Vitamin D and its products and the enzymes controlling the building and remodelling of the bones is thus altered, leading to some problems.

In past years, before coeliac disease was so frequently recognized and properly treated, rickets (**osteomalacia**) occurred, and there were many reports. Fortunately, these are now extremely rare in Western countries. However, 'thinning' of the bones, **osteopenia** or, more severely, osteoporosis, do occur.

It is important to remember that bones naturally become less dense as all people get older. The rate of this effect quickens in women after the menopause. Osteopenia and osteoporosis are defined by the World Health Organization using statistical analysis of thousands of results in normal populations. Hence, osteopenia is the degree of reduced density at the lower end of the range and is defined as being present in about 16 per cent of the population; osteoporosis is more severe, being present in approximately 3 per cent of the population. These percentages increase substantially as people get older. Despite these population figures, very few patients have any noticeable effects from their bone disease. Older people, as we all know, may get shorter and somewhat bent over due to the spine getting less dense and shrinking; they are also prone to fracture a bone more easily if they fall. There are several surveys in coeliac patients showing that slightly more of them have osteopenia and also osteoporosis. This is worse in untreated patients. However, there is very little evidence that they have a significantly increased risk of fracture and we can conclude that the effects of osteoporosis in coeliac patients do not seem to be much greater than those in any person who is getting older.

It is good advice, however, to make sure the coeliac disease is well treated with a strict GFD, since this is certainly helpful to the bones, and that there is an adequate intake of calcium and Vitamin D. If osteoporosis is found on a scan, or a fracture has occurred, specific medication should be considered in conjunction with the patient's doctor. General advice for all people to produce healthy bones includes regular exercise, stopping smoking and reducing the excess intake of alcohol.

Hyposplenism (reduced function of the spleen)

Reduced function of the spleen, which has a mild effect on immune function, does occur in coeliac disease. It is usually detected by finding some unusually shaped blood cells in the circulation, which are old and would normally have been removed by the spleen. It improves to a large extent with a GFD, and there is very little evidence that it has a major clinical effect in patients. There is a theoretical risk of increased pneumococcal infections, but this has not been borne out in practice.

Complications affecting the intestinal mucosa

Refractory coeliac disease

refractory coeliac disease
A very rare form of coeliac disease. The small intestinal mucosa does not improve as expected with a gluten-free diet. This can occur in people already diagnosed some time previously, who begin to deteriorate, or can be found in newly diagnosed patients. The patients can have severe gastrointestinal symptoms and poor nutrition.

Refractory coeliac disease is where patients do not respond to treatment and they remain clinically unwell. As discussed earlier, in some of these patients it was noted that other conditions may be found, or other treatments need to be added. However, there is a residual number of patients who do not respond to treatment, or have responded and then relapsed, and no other conditions are found to explain it. On follow-up biopsy as part of their assessment, the small intestinal mucosa will remain abnormal and typical of coeliac disease. Such patients probably represent about one per cent of the coeliac population. They may continue for many years with less than normal health, but come to no major harm. However, they do have continuing absorption problems and less than adequate nutrition. Specialist follow-up is necessary and, apart from attempting treatment with steroids or immuno-suppressive drugs such as azathioprine, nutritional replacement will be necessary, with special supplements and additional vitamins and minerals. Very occasionally these patients become so malnourished that they require a long period of treatment in hospital with intravenous (through a vein) feeding. A biopsy test in such patients may show the severe Grade 4 features in the mucosa (see Chapter 5).

Medical specialists caring for such patients are always on the look-out for a more serious progression. Hence CT scans are often repeated, barium X-rays are performed and multiple biopsies obtained. Even surgery to look directly at the intestine is sometimes undertaken. All these measures are aimed at discovering whether or not the patient has a malignancy, or ulceration of the small intestine.

my experience

I was diagnosed with coeliac disease 25 years ago, when I was still working as a school secretary. The children had just left home and I was looking forward to having more time to myself. However, I felt so tired when I got home in the evenings that I just flopped down in front of the television. Eventually, through being found to be anaemic, I had a biopsy test and coeliac disease was diagnosed. It was a relief to find there was a cause for my symptoms, and I started a gluten-free diet. I soon got the hang of the diet since I like cooking and began to make all my own bread – even my husband began to eat it!

After about 18 months my consultant suggested I should have another biopsy test – which I didn't relish since, in those days, it involved swallowing a biopsy capsule. However, I thought it was for the best and had it done. The result showed that there was an improvement in the lining of the intestine, but it was not 'normal'; only a 50 per cent improvement the consultant said. However, my anaemia had been cured and I was able to stop the iron tablets. I continued to get very tired though, but overall I was feeling better.

Two years later I had another biopsy test, but this was much easier since they used a new camera endoscope; it was much quicker and was finished before I recovered from the sedative injection. Unfortunately, the biopsy was slightly worse than before. I nearly fell out with the consultant and the dietitian at the hospital, since they thought I wasn't sticking to my gluten-free diet properly. I know they were only trying to make sure about the diet, but it makes you feel so guilty. However, I was sure that my diet was strictly gluten-free, and the dietitian confirmed that when we went through a diet diary I kept for a couple of weeks. My consultant was concerned to help, despite my being cross with him, and explained that perhaps we should investigate further. I was not keen since I did feel better, I had more responsibility at work and, although I felt tired all the time, I felt I was managing well.

Two or three years later, however, I agreed to more tests. I had another endoscopy with a biopsy taken, and also a barium X-ray of my intestines and a CT scan of my body. I had other tests to look for infection in the bowel, how my pancreas was working, whether or not I could eat dairy products and if I had diabetes or thyroid trouble. These involved testing my urine, my blood and my breath. However, all the tests were normal, except for the biopsy which still showed that the lining of my small intestine was virtually no different from when I was first diagnosed. Therefore there had been some initial improvement my consultant said, but then a deterioration. He was sure I had coeliac disease but that it wasn't responding now to a gluten-free diet. I tried a very strict diet, both gluten-free and wheat-free. This didn't help with my tiredness and a later biopsy test showed no improvement. He suggested that I try a course of steroids, but I wasn't keen on that. I had heard of the side-effects. I know, of course, they cause osteoporosis and since I was now past the menopause I didn't want to make my bones worse.

Since then I have seen my consultant every nine to 12 months. He tells me that my condition is very rare, but that I am very interesting! I am still about the same, certainly no worse and, since I have retired, life is quite good. I stick to a strict gluten-free diet and have had two more endoscopic biopsies, both showing what my consultant calls refractory coeliac disease. He is certainly very attentive and has discussed all my biopsies with several biopsy specialists, but he says there is nothing to worry about. He did explain that there may be a risk of some type of cancer, but I haven't got that and he will simply 'keep an eye on me'! Overall, I enjoy life. I am easily tired, but we go away on holiday to see our son in America, and I like gardening. One good result was that despite all my medical history, my bones are no thinner than expected at my age. My consultant was pleased about that.

Ulcerative jejunitis

Very rarely patients with refractory coeliac disease, as described above, or presenting for the very first time as untreated patients, may have severe malabsorption which fails to respond as expected to treatment. They are in a severe clinical condition with dehydration, abdominal pain, diarrhoea and malnutrition. They are found to have not only an abnormal small intestinal mucosa, but also chronic ulcers throughout the jejunum and ileum. They require intravenous feeding, blood transfusion, steroids and azathioprine, and have a poor prognosis, with a high mortality. This condition is called **ulcerative jejunitis**, and most cases of it arise as a complication of coeliac disease. It is very rare.

Small intestinal lymphoma

Close examination of the cells in biopsies from patients with ulcerative jejunitis or refractory coeliac disease can reveal abnormal lymphocytes which are malignant. These multiply and cause a **lymphoma** of the small intestine. The lymphocytes are frequently T cells, so that the

ulcerative jejunitis
A very rare condition in which there are widespread ulcers in the small intestine. This leads to poor intestinal function with weight loss, malnutrition and severe diarrhoea. If it occurs, it is usually a rare complication of coeliac disease. Unfortunately, the outlook is poor.

lymphoma
An uncontrolled multiplication of abnormal lymphocytes within the body, which are usually malignant (i.e. cancerous). Many are found to be circulating in the blood and collect in the lymph nodes, causing them to enlarge where they can be felt.

lymphoma is referred to by specialists as 'enteropathy-associated T-cell lymphoma' (EATL). This type of lymphoma, as in the conditions described above, occurs in known coeliac patients, usually poorly treated, or in new, unknown, cases. Once again, the patients may have severe symptoms of weight loss, abdominal pain, diarrhoea and severe weakness. Alternatively, they may come to hospital as an emergency, with severe abdominal pain due to the fact that an ulcer or tumour (lymphoma) of the small intestine has perforated the intestine. Patients diagnosed with lymphoma in coeliac disease have a poor outlook overall, although nowadays more have been treated with chemotherapy and have received benefit.

It must be stressed that these serious complications of the intestinal mucosa are very rare. There are no accurate figures for the numbers in the coeliac population, although estimates suggest they occur in less than 0.1 per cent (1 in 1000) coeliac patients. There is no doubt, however, that treatment of coeliac patients with a strict GFD reduces the risk of these complications, so that after three to five years on a GFD the risk of these rare conditions is similar to that in the general population. The excess mortality rate reported in coeliac disease is due to the few cases of these rare complications occurring in new or poorly treated patients.

Other malignancies

Apart from malignancy of the lymphocytes (lymphoma), the frequency of other malignancies has been assessed in coeliac patients. There is a slight increase in the number of cancers of the oesophagus and small intestine,

myth
Coeliac disease, because it is permanent and life-long, shortens one's life.

fact
Treated coeliac patients have a normal life expectancy. Surveys show that slightly more untreated coeliac patients than the healthy population die earlier. This is due to a few cases of severe, complicated, untreated coeliac disease. Such cases are very rare. Once treated on a strict gluten-free diet, life expectancy of coeliac patients is normal.

but these are even less common than the rare lymphoma. Interestingly, there is a reduced frequency of breast cancer in women with coeliac disease. Why this is, is unknown.

CHAPTER

7

Taking control: living with coeliac disease

Fortunately, we are all different and this means that we cope with our lives and health issues in a variety of ways. This will depend upon our personality, our upbringing, our age and our personal circumstances. For example, if we have some background in health matters this may make it easier for us to understand and cope with a life-long condition such as coeliac disease. Whatever your circumstances, however, it is hoped this chapter will give you practical ideas about living with the disease.

When the diagnosis is first made, many patients will feel relief that a cause for their symptoms, which may have been present for some time, has been found. They will feel particularly relieved when, as happens in the majority of patients, they begin to feel better on a gluten-free diet. However, some patients may feel angry that they have a life-long condition, or that it has taken a long time to diagnose. This is a normal reaction in some people to any new problem, and health care professionals should understand that. With the passage of time and with sympathetic follow-up and informed dietary advice, such feelings of anger and frustration do improve.

Some patients may go through a phase of denial, particularly those perhaps who are diagnosed incidentally by family screening or in association with another condition such as diabetes. They do not feel ill as a consequence of the condition, and find a GFD irksome. Once again, patient explanation of the condition and of the long-term problems likely to occur without proper dietary treatment are required.

Teenagers

As already hinted at in earlier chapters, many teenagers find it particularly difficult to stick to a GFD. There is a variety of reasons. The sensitivity to gluten seems to decrease in the teenage years and therefore, even if teenagers with coeliac disease eat gluten-containing food, they may have virtually no symptoms. 'Why bother with the diet?' is a question which they ask. The food which teenagers tend to like is often gluten-containing, for example burgers, butties, sauces on takeaways and food fried in batter. Peer pressure to conform is also an important influence in their lives. Teenage rebellion is something which we all felt, whether or not we expressed it! Hence teenage patients need sympathetic and flexible health care and advice.

In my dealings with teenagers, I encourage them to keep attending my coeliac clinic, and am willing to be flexible about appointment dates. I encourage them to be honest about their dietary lapses in a non-judgemental way, so that they feel confident to continue under medical supervision. As they grow older they will then find it easier to discuss such issues as, for example, managing a GFD whilst providing a balanced diet for a family, or the dietary needs during pregnancy, or managing an associated condition as well as coeliac disease.

my experience

I still feel very cross about it all but 'that's life' as my dad is always saying – not that it's any use!

It all started out of the blue four years ago; I had just left sixth form college and was starting a job as a secretary. My dad had bought me a car, I had a great bunch of friends and we went out most evenings. One day I fainted at work. There was a panic and I ended up in the Accident & Emergency department at our local hospital; that was an experience, but that's another story! They said I was very anaemic and I stayed in overnight to have a blood transfusion. Apparently my blood count was only half what it should have been.

I then went to an out-patient clinic and had various blood tests. One came back as positive for coeliac disease. I'd never heard of it, and didn't like the sound of it when the doctor told me about it, and especially the diet – yuk! They said I should have an endoscopy test with a biopsy of my intestine. That sounded awful, but my dad said I should have it; he went on so much that, in the end, I gave in. I made so much fuss I think they must have given me all the sedatives in the hospital but, in fact, I don't remember much about it. The biopsy result showed I had coeliac disease, but I didn't believe it. I was feeling well, and had a new boyfriend. I didn't want to change my diet. How can you when you go out every night?

Eventually, after a lot of nagging from my mum and dad, I tried to follow the gluten-free diet. The dietitian at the hospital tried to help, but it's so boring to go on that diet. When I went to the clinic again, the doctor tried to insist that the diet would be good for me. I said I felt perfectly well without the diet, and I didn't believe I had the disease. We agreed in the end that I would try the diet for about three months, and then see how things were. I did try, but it wasn't easy.

After three months I agreed to have another endoscopy test. This time the biopsy showed some improvement and the doctor said it was fantastic. Well, I didn't think so. I said I was fed up with the diet, I didn't feel any different and if I got anaemic again they could always give me a blood transfusion. That resulted in a big argument at home, as you can guess. Surprisingly, the doctor said it was my decision, my life and he would see me again in a few months, but he was convinced I did have coeliac disease.

Well, we had a great six months. Nigel, my boyfriend, and I moved in together and I started planning a wedding. I missed one hospital appointment, and when I eventually went it was about 12 months later. I had a blood test and my blood count was down again. Not as bad as before, but pretty low. The doctor said I needed some iron tablets and what did I think about the coeliac disease. I still wasn't happy about it, and wasn't sure whether I had it. Funnily enough, I agreed to another biopsy test. The doctor said, if the biopsy was abnormal again, would I then believe him! Sure enough, the biopsy did look worse, which must have been because I was eating a normal diet. I still didn't feel poorly.

Well, we're married now, and I do try to stick to my gluten-free diet as much as possible. The doctor at the hospital is quite patient with me and says the diet will keep me more healthy, especially if I have kids, so I guess I'll stick to it – but I do feel cross about having this disease.

It is interesting that teenage patients who were diagnosed as very young children and who therefore do not remember anything other than a GFD, are often far more confident with their dietary management. They do not find it so difficult to explain their diet to their friends and can more easily resist peer pressure.

It must be stressed that many teenagers cope extremely well with coeliac disease and assume a very responsible attitude to their health. I have many patients who are now starting their first jobs, or who are college or university students, and they are role models for us all on how to cope with, and take control of, their own well-being.

Children

Many children who are diagnosed with coeliac disease are less than two years of age. They, of course, must have a gluten-free diet and follow-up similar to adult patients. Introducing and maintaining a GFD is therefore an important task for their parents or carers, but often not a significant problem for the child. They soon get used to the diet. The parents or carers, however, require dietetic advice and education like all new patients. They also need reassurance about their child's future development and sympathetic advice from the health care team.

Older children who are introduced to the GFD will probably find it quite difficult to get used to; ingenuity and initiative will be required on the part of the parents or carers, and dietitians.

Coeliac UK

In the UK we are very fortunate to have a society for patients, which is probably one of the best national coeliac societies in the world. Coeliac UK was founded more than 35 years ago and was one of the first patient self-help societies. It was set up by two remarkable people, one the mother of coeliac child and the other a coeliac patient who was also the founder of Amnesty

International. Contact details for Coeliac UK are given later, but at this stage it must be remembered by all patients and their parents or carers that the organization is there to provide expert advice and support. Whatever the quality of local health care provision, there is no need to feel isolated and alone. Coeliac UK will provide information and advice about where further help may be available if necessary.

It is easy to feel low or depressed, especially when a long-term disease has been diagnosed, but coeliac disease is a good condition to have if one does have a long-term medical problem, since it can be adequately treated and patients can expect to lead a normal life. A positive outlook on life is to be encouraged – it helps us all!

What can I eat?

A balanced diet for us all – healthy eating

The dietitians at Coeliac UK have summarized six points for a healthy diet, which can apply to us all, whether or not we have coeliac disease.

1 Aim to eat five portions of fruit and vegetables each day.

Fruit and vegetables are high in fibre and low in fat and calories. They are also filling. They are rich in antioxidants, vitamins and minerals which provide health benefits, particularly for cardiovascular disease. They are all gluten-free, whether fresh, frozen, dried or canned.

A portion of fruit and vegetables is:

◇ one medium piece of fruit, for example, an apple
◇ two small pieces of fruit, for example, plums
◇ a small handful of very small fruit, for example, grapes
◇ an individual bowl of salad
◇ three tablespoons of vegetables.

2 Reduce fat intake.

All **fats** are high in calories. *Saturated* fats are found in animal products, including meats and dairy produce. They are used in processed foods such as pastry, biscuits and cakes. These are the fats we should try to reduce in our diet, so we should eat lean meat, remove the skin from poultry and swap full fat dairy products for low fat ones.

Polyunsaturated and *monounsaturated* fats come from vegetables, for example olive oil (monounsaturated) and sunflower oil (polyunsaturated). Polyunsaturates also occur in oily fish (mackerel, salmon, tuna). These are beneficial and restrictions on intake are not necessary.

3 Eat plenty of fibre.

Apart from fruit and vegetables, many cereals which coeliac patients can eat are high fibre **carbohydrates**, being low in fat and calories, for example, buckwheat, corn, brown rice, pulses, chickpea flour, sorghum and polenta. Fibre in the diet helps promote normal bowel function and has an effect on keeping the cholesterol under control.

4 Cut salt intake.

Most people eat too much **salt**, which contributes to high blood pressure and heart

fat
A series of biological compounds made up of different chemicals called fatty acids and glycerol. Fat is used by living organisms as a good way of storing energy (calories) for later use.

carbohydrates
Complex biological compounds containing carbon, hydrogen and oxygen in various combinations. Important in forming the structure of organisms and also, especially in plants, in storing energy (starch) (see Chapter 6).

salt
A common mineral called sodium chloride (NaCl), naturally present in all living organisms and hence all food. It is an essential component of body fluids and is finely balanced by the body. Added to food, it acts as a preservative and enhances the taste, but too much can lead to ill health.

disease. Aim to reduce processed foods and snacks such as crisps and nuts, which are high in salt. One can soon get used to food cooked without salt. Experiment with herbs and spices to add flavouring, and do not add extra salt at the table.

5 Keep a healthy weight.

Being overweight is certainly bad for your health. Proper dietary advice and support is often necessary to lose weight successfully, but it needs a lot of willpower! A balanced diet is important, cutting down on high fat and high sugar foods. Regular exercise, at least 20 minutes walking each day, is also important for good health and weight control.

6 Drink within sensible limits.

Aim to drink at least two litres (three-and-a-half pints) of fluid each day. Most people drink too little. Care should be taken to drink within the safe limits for alcohol, that is two **units** per day for women and three units per day for men (14 units and 21 units per week respectively). One unit is half a pint of cider or gluten-free beer, one small glass of wine, or one measure of spirits. One alcohol-free day each week is good, and don't have all your 14 or 21 units at one time – avoid binge drinking!

It is easy for coeliac patients to be so careful about their GFD that they forget about the need for healthy eating as outlined above. By eating a balanced diet, you will not only avoid becoming overweight but also help to ensure adequate intake of necessary nutrients such as calcium and iron. Seeking advice at the annual check-ups for coeliac patients can be very helpful in this regard.

units of alcohol

These are defined as the equivalent amount of pure alcohol (ethanol) in any particular volume of beverage. This obviously varies with the strength and the type of alcoholic drink. Thus one unit is present in a half pint of 'normal' strength beer or lager, one 'moderate' size glass of wine, or one standard measure of spirits. It is easy to underestimate the amount of alcohol and therefore to drink more than imagined. The recommended safe limits per week are 21 units for men and 14 units for women.

> **Q** I have been on a strict gluten-free diet for several years and regained weight, but now, despite taking only the recommended number of calories, I am still putting on weight. Why?
>
> **A** Your initial increase in weight after starting a gluten-free diet was due to the fact that your small intestinal mucosa was healing and absorbing more nutrition. Your absorption should now be back to normal. You may also have a better appetite than before diagnosis. It may be that you are not using as much energy as you think. More regular daily exercise will help. It is less likely that there is a medical cause for your weight increase, but if you are unwell in any way you should see your doctor. Advice on your weight management should be available from your local dietitian who can assess the calorie intake and healthy balance of your individual diet.

myth
Some people cannot tolerate a gluten-free diet.

fact
Many patients, particularly initially, find a gluten-free diet unusual, or less palatable, until they get used to it. You may feel more hungry as wheat and gluten-containing cereals that are part of a normal diet are more sustaining than gluten-free cereals like rice. However, there is usually no obvious reason why some people seem unable to tolerate a gluten-free diet (apart from those who have lactose intolerance, which is explained later in this chapter).

In my experience, there is sometimes some confusion about our daily calcium needs. The normal daily adult requirement is about 750 mg, but it is recommended that coeliac patients should have twice that, especially in the early years after diagnosis in adults, or in growing teenagers. It may be difficult to get 1500 mg (that is 2 x 750 mg) from the diet, and so calcium supplement tablets are usually recommended. These are important in helping you to achieve calcium requirements for good bone health but missing an odd dose will not be detrimental.

Foods rich in calcium include milk (full fat or skimmed), cheese, yoghurt and sardines. A pint of milk contains approximately 700 mg calcium.

> **Q** Should all coeliac patients take calcium tablets?
>
> **A** It is not necessary for all patients. However, adequate calcium intake is important. Many patients will get sufficient calcium from their diet,

A particularly if they have plenty of milk and dairy products. If a bone scan (DEXA) has suggested the bones are less dense (osteopenia or osteoporosis), many doctors would recommend taking combined calcium and Vitamin D tablets daily. It is best to use prescribed calcium tablets in recommended doses as some over-the-counter products do not have sufficient calcium levels. This should be discussed with your dietitian or doctor.

Daily energy requirements

Although it is important to eat a balanced diet, it is also important to know how much we need each day. The average requirements to provide the energy we need are measured in **calories** (kcals). The estimated average requirements for children and adults are shown in Table 6. It is recommended that half (50 per cent) of this energy intake is in the form of carbohydrate which, in the UK, is mainly derived from cereals. Hence it is important for the coeliac patient to understand clearly which cereals or alternative sources of carbohydrate can be eaten.

calorie content
The amount of energy produced from each gram of a particular food when used by the body for normal functioning. A minimum and maximum number is required each day, depending upon age and activity, to keep healthy.

Table 6 Estimated average energy requirements per day for males and females at different ages.

Age (years)	Male (kcals/day)	Female (kcals/day)
1–3	1230	1165
4–6	1715	1545
7–10	1970	1740
11–14	2220	1845
15–18	2755	2110
19–49	2550	1940
50–59	2550	1900
60–64	2380	1900
65–74	2330	1900
75+	2100	1810

my experience

I was diagnosed with dermatitis herpetiformis three years ago. This involved having a biopsy test of the intestine, and I was told that this also showed the abnormality of coeliac disease. Although my rash improved a lot with the dapsone tablets, I was strongly advised to go on a gluten-free diet. I must say this has helped my skin enormously, and I do feel much fitter.

The gluten-free diet made quite a change to my life, however. I think I was fortunate in having a very helpful dietitian at the local hospital. She saw me within two to three weeks of the diet being recommended. The first thing she did was to reassure me that my condition was not dangerous and that since it would take some time to get used to the gluten-free diet, I could expect to make some mistakes. She also reassured me that making mistakes would not be dangerous, but they were best avoided if possible.

At our first appointment, she told me a bit about the gluten-free diet and then went through my own diet to see what sort of changes should be made. That was quite interesting, since the most challenging meal was breakfast. I always had cornflakes and toast with marmalade. Now I have rice crispies or other rice-based cereals, and gluten-free bread toasted, still with my homemade marmalade. I have got used to this and it suits me fine. She did recommend grapefruit and eggs cooked in various ways, but I only have those when we stay in an hotel. Lunch and evening meals were much less of a problem. We always like various meats and fish, and have plenty of vegetables, potatoes or rice. Gluten-free pasta is now very good – you can hardly tell the difference from normal pasta and we have always been fond of salads too. Milk puddings, jellies and fruit are good to choose when away from home. When I'm feeling enthusiastic there are some wonderful gluten-free puddings to make from the various gluten-free recipe books.

There is a variety of snacks which are OK to eat – not only my homemade cakes, but gluten-free fruit and nut bars, yoghurts, fruit and sandwiches with gluten-free rolls. It's surprising how many sandwich fillings can be gluten-free.

The dietitian also gave me some diet sheets to study, some details about joining Coeliac UK and some starter packs of gluten-free samples from different food manufacturers. That seemed a lot to take in at once! However, I arranged to see the dietitian again after two to three months. By that time I was beginning to manage quite well. The Coeliac UK Food and Drink Directory is extremely valuable while shopping, as is their telephone helpline. The dietitian worked out with me what gluten-free food I would need on prescription, and she contacted my GP's surgery to suggest what my monthly prescription should be. That was very helpful, since it was only the dietitian who really seemed to know what I would need. After the first month I decided to invest in a pre-paid prescription certificate which, although expensive at first, has saved quite a lot over 12 months.

I saw the dietitian after six months on the diet, and she said I was doing fine. By that time she had also assessed my calcium and iron needs, and made various recommendations to increase them in my diet. I have now arranged to see her just once a year when I go to the follow-up clinic at the hospital.

I can truly say that although the gluten-free diet has made a big change to my life, once I got the hang of it, it is not too bad and I feel much better overall. My dermatitis herpetiformis rash has also completely gone, and I have stopped the dapsone tablets now. It's a great relief to get rid of the itching!

A gluten-free diet

In getting started on a gluten-free diet, the patient must first remember what can be eaten: all fresh meat, poultry, fish, dairy products, fruit and vegetables, which will provide a lot of nutrients and variety to the diet. Foods containing gluten, however, are to be avoided, which normally means bread, flour, cakes, pastries and biscuits. Many manufactured gluten-free alternatives are available in the shops and products available on prescription in the UK (FP10 from your GP) are:

◇ bread loaves and rolls
◇ plain biscuits
◇ crackers and crispbreads
◇ flour and flour-type mixes
◇ pasta
◇ pizza bases.

The problem for new patients and carers in learning about a gluten-free diet is in knowing where gluten may be found, since wheat flour is widely used in processed foods – sometimes in surprising places! Frequently overlooked foods that often contain gluten include: baked beans, chocolate bars, communion wafers, dry roasted nuts, gravy, meatloaf, salad dressings, sauces, sausages, soups, soy sauce and stuffing.

Of course, there are varieties of the above which are gluten-free, hence you will have to read the food labels carefully and consult the Coeliac UK Food and Drink Directory. Coeliac UK has a good introductory leaflet called 'Getting Started: Gluten-free Check List' which summarizes very well which products can and cannot be eaten, and what needs checking. It is available free of charge to members of Coeliac UK (see 'Further Help' section at the end of the book).

Food labelling is now very helpful. Gluten, wheat or related compounds must be listed either clearly in the ingredients list or in an 'Allergen Advice' box on a food label if they are used as ingredients. If gluten, wheat or barley is not highlighted as being present in the product, it means the product is safe for people with coeliac disease. The crossed grain symbol is a useful tool to denote safe eating for people with coeliac disease. It is owned by Coeliac UK and used under licence by food manufacturers whose products comply with the gluten-free standard.

Names are confusing and sometimes food manufactures can use ingredients that sound like they contain gluten when they are, in fact, gluten-free. Examples of these includes:

- ✧ Maize starch
- ✧ Modified starch
- ✧ Modified maize starch
- ✧ Maltodextrin
- ✧ Glucose syrup
- ✧ Sorbitol
- ✧ Maltitol
- ✧ Isomalt
- ✧ Textured vegetable protein
- ✧ Caramel
- ✧ Artificial sweetener
- ✧ Aspartame
- ✧ Dextrose
- ✧ Xantham gum

Some ingredients which are used in food manufacture do contain gluten and should be checked on the food label. These include wheat starch, modified wheat starch, malt and barley flour. (See Chapter 6 for the safety of Codex wheat starch.) Coeliac UK's Food and Drink Directory contains a check list of gluten-containing and gluten-free ingredients.

Dietary mistakes

Coeliac patients can expect to make mistakes from time to time, and to eat something which contains gluten. This is particularly likely when newly diagnosed or when trying to vary the diet with new ideas. It is important not to panic if you find you have eaten something containing gluten. It may be that you will get no symptoms at all, or perhaps some mild gastrointestinal symptoms over 24 hours. Patients often worry that they will damage the lining of the intestine so much that all the good work from taking a GFD will be lost! This is not the case and, although some change may occur with inadvertent gluten ingestion, healing quickly takes place once a GFD is strictly adhered to again. Thus a lapse in the diet is unlikely to do lasting damage to the intestinal mucosa.

Whilst it is true that we all make mistakes from time to time, it has to be said that the ability to stick to a GFD with less mistakes or lapses is helped by regular follow-up and contact with the health care team, especially the experienced dietitian.

Prescriptions

Once a diagnosis of coeliac disease or dermatitis herpetiformis has been made, a patient is entitled to receive some everyday gluten-free foods on prescription (see p. 120). This can help with sticking to the diet and can be cheaper than buying them elsewhere.

When first diagnosed, a patient will clearly require a lot of discussion with their GP or practice dietitian and/or pharmacist. An estimate will have to be made about how much bread, pasta and biscuits is normally eaten in a month, and the dietitian will need to check if this is the correct amount for age and sex, taking into account one's expected energy requirements, as set out in Table 6. Once the amounts are agreed, most GPs renew the prescriptions automatically on a monthly basis, but you will need to give good notice, especially since the pharmacist may need to order the products.

Table 7 Prescribable gluten-free foods.

Food item	Units
400 gm bread/rolls/baguettes	1
500 gm bread/flour/cake mix	2
200 gm sweet/savoury biscuits/crackers/crispbreads	1
250 gm pasta	1
2 pizza bases	1

Table 8 Minimum monthly gluten-free food prescription requirements.

Age and sex	Units per month
Male and female 1–3 years	10
Male and female 4–6 years	11
Male and female 7–10 years	13
Male and female 11–14 years	15
Male and female 15–18 years	18
Male 19–59 years	18
Male 60–74 years	16
Male 75+ years	14
Female 19–74 years	14
Female 75+ years	12
Breast feeding	Add 4
Last third of pregnancy	Add 1
High physical activity	Add 4

The British Dietetic Association, Coeliac UK and the Primary Care Society for Gastroenterology have supported the production of a Prescribing Guide for gluten-free products. This gives recommendations for the minimum monthly gluten-free prescription requirements for various patient groups based on their nutritional needs. The requirements are in a number of units of food items per month. Table 7 shows the number of units represented by each prescribable food item.

Table 8 lists the monthly *minimum* recommended units, depending upon age and sex.

The food examples given can be interchanged, for example bread mixes can be interchanged for rolls, or loaves. Thus, in the case of a male patient, aged 19–59 years, the recommended number of units of prescribable gluten-free food is a minimum of 18. These 18 units could be made up of ten x 400 gm loaves of bread (or five x 500 gm mixes suitable for making bread) (i.e. 10 units), two pizza bases (1 unit), 500 gm pasta (2 units), two x 200 gm crackers (2 units), 200 gm sweet biscuits (1 unit) and 500 gm flour mix (2 units).

Payment for prescriptions

Unless you qualify for free prescriptions for some reason, you will be required to pay the prescription charge for each type of gluten-free food. To save money, it will be beneficial to buy a pre-payment certificate for four or 12 months. Your pharmacist can advise about payment or entitlement to free prescriptions, or you can find out more from the Department of Health website (see 'Further Help'). For a pre-payment certificate, form FP95 is required. Your pharmacist should have some.

Q I was talking to a friend who has coeliac disease and I put myself on a gluten-free diet. It has certainly helped with some abdominal discomfort and bloating I have. My GP will not prescribe gluten-free products. Why?

A Your GP can only prescribe specific treatment for a particular disease. Clearly you have not had coeliac disease diagnosed, according to current recommended criteria. You may have coeliac disease, but we do not know. Your GP cannot prescribe gluten-free products in such a situation. You should discuss it with him/her and seek to make a definite diagnosis of coeliac disease, or not.

Cooking and preparing food

Having obtained supplies of gluten-free food, and consulted the food labels and the Coeliac UK Food and Drink Directory, you are all set to prepare some meals!

Of course, it is the cereal products which are the challenge. Any food which usually contains wheat, barley or rye flour has to be made with alternative ingredients. Most everyday meals and snacks can be prepared with gluten-free products. The special gluten-free flours now available are the result of a great deal of research and development by the manufacturers, and have vastly improved in recent years. Using these flours to bake cakes and biscuits produces some very good results indeed. It must be said, however, that the good and palatable wheat-free bread it is now possible to bake is not like ordinary bread. This is not surprising, since it is because of wheat's glutinous qualities that it has been bred over thousands of years in order to make bread. You cannot expect a loaf to have quite the same taste or texture without gluten.

Baking cakes, biscuits, bread and pastry requires a fresh approach, and a period of trial and error before you will be happy with the results. Although many people enjoy making their own bread, gluten-free loaves are available, which have improved greatly in quality in recent years. White and brown bread mixes are also available. Gluten-free cookbooks offer useful advice to help you get started. They give advice on the combinations of flours which can be used, and they have good ideas about a wide variety of recipes.

Here are some useful tips for food preparation, on what to do and what not to do:

DO: – use alternative flours, including those made from rice, corn, tapioca, chickpea, buckwheat, potato, soya or millet

– try using Xantham gum in baking – it provides structure and elasticity rather like gluten

– use a variety of naturally gluten-free foods, for example, try adding pulses and root vegetables like sweet potatoes to soups or casseroles

– wash down surfaces and hands before preparing, to cut down on contamination risk

DON'T: – use the same utensils for gluten-containing and gluten-free food, e.g. toasters, breadboards, serving plates, cutlery, deep-fat fryers (which may contain batter) and colanders.

These tips are to improve the quality of your diet and to reduce contamination of gluten-free foods with traces of gluten.

The coeliac lifestyle: living with a gluten-free diet

It is important to stress that, once treated, coeliac patients can lead an entirely normal working and social life, apart from the restrictions of diet. Since much of our lives revolve around eating, drinking and socializing it is only to be expected that some coeliac patients find this very challenging when they change to a gluten-free diet. Even in the pub you may have to change your normal drink and snack. However, it is important to have a positive attitude and not to let your coeliac disease dominate everything, since you will be healthy once the condition is treated properly.

Eating out

Having to eat away from home is worrying, especially when you are going to new places. Knowledge of the gluten-free diet and some self-confidence in describing your needs are important assets in these situations. There is no reason why you should not enjoy meals out, as you have always done. You simply need to take extra precautions and to relay your dietary requirements carefully.

At work

Once familiar with your needs, a works canteen can provide gluten-free meals. Otherwise, like many non-coeliac people, you may have to take a packed lunch (see section below on children's food).

Restaurants

When planning a meal out, it is best to ring the restaurant beforehand to explain your needs. It is vital to have their reassurance that they will take great care to avoid contamination with gluten-containing foods. If explained properly, many chefs are pleased to help and even cook something which is not on the normal menu. In some restaurants you will actually find a menu note to say that the chief understands the GFD and will prepare suitable dishes. If you have to choose from the ordinary menu, avoid soups (unless they are clear). Plainly cooked meats and fish without gravy or sauce are fine. Fish cooked in batter is not suitable (even if you remove the

Q Can I drink lager or shandy?

A Lager and shandy are both made from barley, like other beers. They will contain small amounts of gluten, even though in shandy it will be more dilute. You should therefore avoid them or have one of the gluten-free beers now available.

myth
Beers are alright for coeliac patients.

fact
Until recently, all beers were made from barley and contained varying amounts of gluten. Some beers are now available which are gluten-free, so they are alright to drink. Alternatives are cider, wines and spirits (all in moderation!).

batter, the fish will still be contaminated with gluten). Salads are safe, but dressings may contain gluten. Unfortunately, many tempting puddings contain gluten, although fruit, fruit salad, sorbet and cheese are all fine.

Takeaways and fast food

These can be more difficult for the coeliac patient. Fortunately, more and more fish and chip shops and cafés are starting to make gluten-free batter, and will cook fish and chips in separate oil which has not been used for frying ordinary batter. You will usually need to ask for chips not to be fried in the same oil as battered fish.

With Chinese food, avoid egg noodles but rice noodles and plain rice are safe. Soy sauce contains wheat and therefore should be avoided. Unfortunately, contamination is a risk since often Chinese foods are stir-fried in a wok. Some varieties of Japanese Tamari gluten-free soy sauce are available.

With Indian food, avoid all bread. Poppadums are made with chickpea flour, as are many other Indian dishes, so they are gluten-free and should be safe but may be deep-fried in oil that has cooked other battered foods.

When considering Italian food, normal pizza is unsuitable. Some outlets now make gluten-free pizza bases, or will cook toppings on your own gluten-free ones if you take them with you. Several Italian restaurants now make gluten-free pasta, so there may be one near you.

Contamination risk and identification of ingredients in dishes are the main concerns when eating out, or eating on the hoof. If in doubt, you should ask. Some fast-food chains are listed in the Coeliac UK Food and Drink Directory. They do have gluten-free options and are willing to provide more choice.

myth
Occasional takeaways do no harm.

fact
Many takeaways can be gluten-free, but gluten may be present, for example, in some burgers or sausages or batter. If gluten is present, there may be no symptoms after eating the takeaway, but there will be some effects on the small intestinal mucosa. Persistent consumption will produce more major abnormalities. It is better to avoid takeaways if you are not sure whether they contain gluten.

Hotels

Obviously it is important to ring beforehand to explain your gluten-free requirements. Many hotels have no problem in providing what you need. You may have to take some of your own bread and cereal. More and more hotels and guest houses are now advertising as being willing to provide for guests with coeliac disease.

Hospitals

We all may have to be a hospital patient from time to time. Sadly, some hospitals find it difficult to provide gluten-free food immediately. Obviously you should let the ward know beforehand if your admission is pre-arranged. It will be more difficult in an emergency. Many hospital staff will not know what coeliac disease is. You will need to be firm but patient and bringing in your own bread and cereals will be helpful to begin with. The hospital dietitian should be told you are there, so that they can check on the arrangements for your GFD.

Flying

Airlines will sometimes provide gluten-free meals, but will require several days' warning. It is advisable to pack some gluten-free snacks for the flight, just in case!

Keeping healthy

During the last two chapters you have been given a lot of information and advice about the treatment of coeliac disease. All this is to try to keep you as healthy as possible. To summarize, there are some points worth stressing:

✧ Remember that most of the time you will feel well.
✧ Try to stick to a gluten-free diet as strictly as possible
✧ Take regular exercise.
✧ Do not smoke.
✧ Drink enough fluid, but keep alcohol within recommended limits.
✧ Keep in regular contact with the health care team.
✧ Have regular dietetic reviews.
✧ Become a member of Coeliac UK and benefit from the support and information they provide.

Planning a family

Pregnancy and fertility

In well-treated coeliac women, fertility and pregnancy are no different from those without coeliac disease, and female patients should follow the normal advice and routine. It is important to maintain adequate calcium intake and the extra food requirements necessary (see Table 8, p. 123). Folic acid supplements are recommended for all women who are trying to conceive, since in the early months of pregnancy folic acid helps to prevent nervous system damage in the foetus (the most common of which is spina bifida). Iron supplements may also be necessary. Clearly, advice will be available from the ante-natal clinic and the dietitian.

In patients who are untreated or poorly treated for coeliac disease, there is a slightly increased risk of miscarriage, of infertility and of a low birth weight baby. Dietary lapses can, potentially, lead to reduced absorption of nutrients and can thus affect the baby's growth. The message is clear: a strict gluten-free diet leads to healthy mothers and healthy babies. The vast majority of coeliac mothers do have entirely normal pregnancies and healthy children.

Weaning

Since coeliac disease runs in families, parents with coeliac disease worry that their baby may have the condition. There is a one in ten chance of this, which means that nine out of ten babies will not have coeliac disease. Most children who develop coeliac disease do not have a family history of the condition.

There is some evidence that delaying the introduction of cereals and gluten-containing foods, and prolonging breast feeding, helps to delay or even prevent coeliac disease developing in any child (whether from coeliac parents or not). It is probably sensible, therefore, not to introduce solids before the age of six months if possible, while continuing some breast feeding. However, introduction of solids may occur from four months. If weaning is commenced before the age of six months any food given should be gluten-free until the baby has reached six months. Ready-made baby foods for those up to six months of age are gluten-free, and the first solid foods should include pureed fruit, vegetables and baby rice – all of which are gluten-free. At eight or nine months the baby can start eating normal foods such as bread, pasta, cereals and puddings. Obviously advice from the dietitian and health visitor is very important.

Other medical conditions and situations

Diabetes

It has already been mentioned that Type 1 diabetes and coeliac disease may occur in the same patient. This happens in about six per cent of diabetic patients. Usually the diabetes is diagnosed first. It is clearly a dietary challenge. With a gluten-free diet it is possible to maintain a balanced diet and to have a regular carbohydrate intake to help with blood glucose control. A high fibre intake also helps, but this can be more difficult for coeliac patients. They should eat plenty of fruit and vegetables. For breakfast they should have brown rice breakfast cereals, buckwheat flakes and gluten-free muesli with added dried fruit, nuts and seeds. Gluten-free pasta, brown rice and polenta are useful for main meals. Pulses should be added to casseroles and salads.

Dermatitis herpetiformis

These patients should be treated similarly to those with coeliac disease, since they have the same small intestinal abnormality. The skin condition often requires drug treatment as well, at least initially. The most commonly used drug is dapsone, but this must be taken under medical supervision (see Chapter 4).

Osteoporosis

Much has already been included about osteoporosis. Remember the importance of adequate calcium and Vitamin D intake, regular exercise, not smoking and sensible drinking. Drug treatment is available as well if osteoporosis has developed. In that case, DEXA scanning for follow-up will be required.

Vegetarians

People who are vegetarians, and particularly those who do not eat dairy produce or eggs (vegans) are at greater risk of developing nutritional deficiencies. This is because the vegan diet in particular restricts intake of the prime sources of calcium, Vitamin B_{12} and iron. Many fruits and vegetables do contain these vitamins and minerals, but absorption is more efficient from animal sources so it may be difficult to get adequate amounts purely from a vegetarian gluten-free diet. Supplements of calcium, iron, folic acid and Vitamin B_{12} may therefore be needed.

Lactose intolerance

Lactose is the type of sugar present in milk from humans, cows, sheep and goats. It is digested by the **enzyme** lactase in our small intestine. When

enzyme
A biological chemical which effects reactions within the cells.

this enzyme is deficient, the symptoms of lactose intolerance can occur. These include nausea, bloating, diarrhoea and abdominal discomfort. It is very common worldwide, and the norm in those of non-European ancestry. In European adults it occurs in up to 30 per cent of people, but does not always cause symptoms. The treatment is to avoid milk and milk products, although it is frequently only necessary to reduce these rather than exclude them totally.

In coeliac disease, because the small intestine is abnormal when untreated, lactose intolerance may also be present although this is usually temporary. It normally improves as the villi re-grow while the patient is taking the GFD. However, if a reduced lactose diet is also necessary the calcium intake will need to be maintained in some other way. Dietary advice is clearly necessary. It is reassuring to know that lactose intolerance is not a problem in the vast majority of treated coeliac patients in the UK.

Insurance

There should be no difficulty in obtaining life or travel insurance. Insurance companies will require a medical report from your doctor, and they may increase the premiums slightly in the early years after diagnosis, but after four or five years of good health these will usually be the same as for people without coeliac disease.

It is important to get advice from a proper financial adviser or insurance broker. Telephone advice can often be rigid and not able to deal flexibly with specific issues like coeliac disease and its treatment. Coeliac UK has some general information on this topic.

Situations involving children

It will be apparent from earlier chapters that in children coeliac disease can be diagnosed particularly at a young age soon after weaning. They, of course, must have a gluten-free diet and follow-up similar to adult patients. It is important that children with coeliac disease grow and develop normally, and with proper treatment there should be no problems. Earlier in this chapter the energy requirements and units of gluten-free food for prescriptions were summarized showing the amounts necessary at different ages (see Tables 6, 7 and 8, pp. 117, 123). As already mentioned, older children and teenagers may have some personal difficulties in recognizing the need for long-term treatment of their condition, and patience on all sides is required!

Why some patients develop recognizable disease as children and others as adults is unknown. We do know that, in retrospect, 30 per cent of adult patients do appear to have had symptoms as children, which could have been due to coeliac disease.

There are some special circumstances for children in which a few specific issues should be mentioned.

> **myth**
> Coeliac children should avoid strenuous physical activity.

> **fact**
> Children with well-treated coeliac disease should be as healthy and fit as any others. Exercise is good for children. Very active children will need enough calories and they might need to increase the gluten-free prescription for foods. Obviously soon after the diagnosis and when treatment is being established, children may have less energy than normal. Coeliac disease is not a good excuse to avoid games lessons at school!

Playgroups and nurseries

Starting to attend a nursery or playgroup is a big step for your child. Obviously you will want things to go well. Beforehand, it is important to see the head of the group and the staff to explain about coeliac disease and a GFD. One can be reassuring that mistakes with the diet are not life-threatening, but that it really is important to avoid them.

For snack time, you will probably have to provide gluten-free snacks for your child (which should be stored separately). Encourage your child to choose milk to drink, since it is an important nutritious drink. Obviously meals have to be gluten-free and you will need to check this carefully with the staff, or provide your own. It is possible to provide good packed lunches (see below). Children do swap food, so the staff will need to be more aware what your child can and cannot eat.

Many young children like playing with types of playdough. Such commercial products can contain gluten, but Coeliac UK has a very good DIY recipe which keeps for several months.

Starting school

The same principles apply as for nurseries and playgroups. Fortunately, as your child gets older, he or she will begin to understand very well what should and shouldn't be eaten.

Before your child starts school, you should arrange to see the head teacher and class teacher to explain about coeliac disease. Schools do not have to provide gluten-free meals, but some school kitchens or meal services will be very helpful. However, we all recognize how difficult organizing these things can be. You may prefer to provide packed lunches for your child.

Packed lunches

All coeliac patients, young and old, require a packed lunch from time to time. They can be very nutritious and help to provide the daily recommendations of fruit and vegetables. Some of the new fresh gluten-free breads, or those made from bread mixes, are suitable for sandwiches. Gluten-free rolls and pitta breads are also worth trying. There is a wide range of gluten-free fillings which can be used such as: egg, cheese, ham, chicken, bacon, tuna, sardines, marmite, jam, GF chocolate spread, GF cheese spread, cream cheese, cottage cheese, salmon, prawns or GF peanut butter.

Other snacks worth trying, especially for children, include sausages, chicken nuggets and fish fingers, all of which are available in a gluten-free alternative. Clearly fresh fruit, vegetables and dried fruit can be important additions to a packed lunch. Puddings or sweets which are available gluten-free include fromage frais, yoghurt, rice pudding, custard, jelly, mousse, fruit bars, rice cakes, cereal bars and chocolate bars.

School activities

If your child attends Breakfast Clubs or After School Clubs, you will need to make similar arrangements to those outlined, and similar snacks or packed meals will have to be provided.

School trips or holidays can be a worry. If your child is keen to go, you will obviously want to encourage them as much as possible. Clearly, the dietary needs will have to be explained beforehand. It is always important to give your child 'emergency' supplies, such as some gluten-free biscuits, crackers or fruit bars. On day trips, all children usually take packed lunches, but it is important that your child knows what food and drink can and cannot be bought in shops and from vending machines.

Making food at school shouldn't be a problem. In fact, understanding a gluten-free diet could be an important part of a food technology curriculum. The main issue is avoiding swallowing any normal flour which may be used in the class. Breathing flour in the air is not a problem, but inhaled flour can be swallowed with saliva, which could be important. Some children wear masks for this type of class, but it can make them embarrassed and it might be easier to avoid such classroom activities. Explaining and discussing with the teacher is important.

Children's parties

It is important that children with coeliac disease are not made to feel 'odd' and you should try hard to make sure that they do not miss out on social activities. Most children like a party, and you should encourage your child to go to friends' parties, or have one themselves. Checking with the organizer about the food is important, but you can provide suitable gluten-free alternatives, which other children may like too, for example, gluten-free chicken nuggets, cocktail sausages, bread, crisps and fairy cakes!

We have already described eating from take-aways or in fast-food restaurants. It is possible to have gluten-free foods from Chinese, Indian, Italian and English outlets.

A final word about children

It is important to stress that almost all children with coeliac disease grow up normally. They become healthy adults leading normal lives. It is very unusual to suffer any psychological effects from feeling 'different'. It is important, however, to help them as they grow and develop not to feel an outsider and to give them self-confidence in managing their diet and lifestyle. It is probably true to say that any problems they have are more likely to be related to other factors than coeliac disease.

It is important to attend follow-up appointments with the heath care team, particularly while they are growing. Busy teenagers find this irksome, but an understanding approach has already been recommended above.

Much good material is provided by Coeliac UK, which forms the basis of some of this chapter. In the Coeliac UK pack for 'Parents and carers' there are many good ideas and suggestions, including a sample letter about coeliac disease which can be sent to your child's new school.

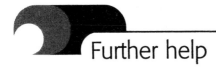

Further help

Useful addresses

Coeliac UK
Suites A–D
Octagon Court
High Wycombe
Bucks HP11 2HS
Tel: 0870 444 8804 (helpline)
Website: www.coeliac.org.uk

Coeliac UK is the patient-based organization which is a national charity for people with coeliac disease and dermatitis herpetiformis. It provides support and a wide range of information for patients, their carers and families.

British Dietetic Association (BDA)
5th Floor, Charles House
148/149 Charles Street
Queensway
Birmingham B3 3HT
Tel: 0121 200 8080
Website: www.bda.uk.com

Department of Health
(information about prescription costs)
Tel: 0845 850 0030
Website: www.dh.gov.uk

Manufacturers and suppliers of gluten-free foods

(Several of these have information centres and helplines.)

Glutafin
(Coeliac Disease Resource Centre)
Nutricia Dietary Care
Newmarket Avenue
White Horse Business Park
Trowbridge
Wilts BA14 0XQ
Careline Tel: 01225 711 801
Website(s): www.glutafin.co.uk
www.trufree.co.uk
email: glutenfree@nutricia.co.uk

Gluten Free Foods Ltd.
Unit 270, Centennial Park
Elstree, Borehamwood
Herts WD6 3SS
Tel: 020 8953 4444
Fax: 020 8953 8285
Website: www.glutenfree-foods.co.uk

Juvela, SHS International
100 Wavertree Boulevard
Liverpool L7 9PT
Advice line: 0151 228 1992
Website: www.juvela.co.uk
email: juvela@shsint.co.uk

Lifestyle Healthcare Ltd
Centenary Business Park
Henley on Thames
Oxfordshire RG9 1DS

Tel: 01491 570 000
Fax: 01491 570 001
Website: www.gfdiet.com
email: sales@gfdiet.com

Nutrition Point Ltd
13 Taurus Park
Westbrook
Warrington WA5 7ZT
Tel: 07041 544 044
(customer care)
Fax: 07041 544 055
Website(s):
www.nutritionpoint.co.uk
www.dietaryspecials.co.uk
email: info@nutritionpoint.co.uk

It is well worth exploring the Coeliac UK website to see the list of publications and the list of suppliers of gluten-free foods, which is quite extensive.

Gluten-free cookery books

Gluten-Free Food, Lyndel Costain and Joanna Farrow, Hamlyn (ISBN 0-600-60793-3).
Healthy Gluten-Free Eating, Darina Allen and Rosemary Kearney, Kyle Cathie Ltd (ISBN 1-85626-542-0).
The Ultimate Gluten-Free Diet, Peter Rawcliffe and Ruth James, Vermilion (ISBN 0-09-188774-7).

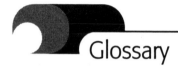

Glossary

Absorption The transfer of food constituents from the lumen (i.e. the hollow centre) of the small intestine, across the epithelium and into the body, for use as nutrition and energy.

Albumin A protein in the blood made by the liver.

Amino acid A basic chemical building block in biology. There are 20 amino acids which are common throughout nature. When they are combined together in various sequences, they form proteins.

Anaemia Present when there is a reduced level of haemoglobin. Haemoglobin is the red chemical, in the red blood cells, which carries oxygen to all parts of the body.

Antibody A specific immunoglobulin molecule directed against a particular substance (an 'antigen').

Antigen A foreign substance, mainly protein, against which an antibody is specifically made by one's own body. Very occasionally the substance against which the antibody is made is not 'foreign' but part of the body itself (this is then an auto-antigen).

Antigen-presenting cell A cell of the immune system involved in initiating an immune reaction. It sticks (presents) an antigen on its surface in order to stimulate a lymphocyte to react.

Atypical coeliac disease Patients with coeliac disease whose symptoms are not obviously gastrointestinal, for example they are diagnosed because of anaemia.

Autoimmune disease A disease in which the body's immune system reacts against its own antigens as if they were foreign.

Bacterium (plural, bacteria) A microscopic organism which causes infection.

Barley A similar plant to wheat; its seeds are grown for food and also for the production of alcoholic drinks (beers, lagers).

Biopsy A small piece of tissue taken for laboratory examination to help with diagnosis or assessment of treatment.

Bone scan (DEXA scan) A type of X-ray scanning which measures the density of the bones.

Calorie content The amount of energy produced from each gram of a particular food when used by the body for normal functioning. A minimum and maximum number is required each day, depending upon age and activity, to keep healthy.

Carbohydrates Complex biological compounds containing carbon, hydrogen and oxygen in various combinations. Important in forming the structure of organisms and also, especially in plants, as storing energy (starch) (see Chapter 6).

Cereal A plant of the grass family which has been developed through evolution and plant breeding to produce seeds which are used as food.

Classical coeliac disease	Patients who have the expected symptoms of coeliac disease, related to the abnormal intestine, for example diarrhoea, weight loss.
Codex wheat starch	Wheat starch which, after milling, is only permitted to have a very small amount of gluten remaining, as laid down by an international standard, and is therefore able to be eaten by most coeliac patients.
Colitis	An inflammation of the large intestine, that is the colon. Symptoms produced include diarrhoea, which may contain blood.
Colon	The last part of the intestinal tract, also called the large intestine; it is about 1.5 metres long and joins the small intestine to the anus (the back passage).
Crypt	A crevice in the mucosa between villi, where the epithelium develops.
CT Scan	A CT (computerized tomography) scan is a series of detailed X-rays taken by a scanning machine, which are then put together by a computer to give detailed pictures of the part of the body which is scanned.
Dapsone	A frequently used medication for dermatitis herpetiformis.
Dermatitis herpetiformis (DH)	A skin condition which has itchy blisters typically on the arms, buttocks and knees. Patients almost all have the small intestinal abnormality of coeliac disease.
DEXA scan	A type of X-ray scanning which measures the density of the bones.
Diabetes	A disease in which there is a high blood in sugar level due to a reduction of, or lack of response to, the hormone insulin from the pancreas. Type 1 diabetes usually occurs in younger people and they require insulin injections for treatment. Type 2 occurs in older, often overweight, people and usually can be treated with tablets.

Digestion	The liquidization and breakdown, within the lumen (i.e. the hollow centre) of the intestine, of food into smaller parts by specific chemicals (enzymes) produced by the body. This enables it to be absorbed into the body for nutrition and energy.
DNA (deoxyribose nucleic acid)	The chemical which is used by the body to make up our genes.
DQ2/DQ8	The symbol of two particular tissue types which are inherited via specific genes. They are present in virtually all coeliac patients, but also in about 30 per cent of non-coeliac people.
Duodenum	The first part of the small intestine, just past the stomach.
EMA	Endomysial antibody. An antibody, usually made of immunoglobulin A by the body, which reacts against an antigen called endomysium, which is a body tissue. The antibody is made almost only by people who have coeliac disease.
Endoscope	A flexible fibre-optic instrument used to examine the inside of the gastrointestinal tract. It is passed through the mouth in order to see the oesophagus (gullet), stomach and duodenum (upper part of the small intestine). A moving television picture of the inside of these organs is seen.
Enterocyte	A cell of the small intestinal epithelium which specializes in absorbing food constituents.
Enteropathy	A disease affecting the intestine.
Enteroscope	An endoscope which is longer than normal. It is made so that it can reach further down into the small intestine. It is more difficult to manipulate than the usual endoscope.
Enzyme	A biological chemical which effects reactions within the cells.
Epithelium	The layer of cells which covers the inside surface of the intestine.

Fat	A series of biological compounds made up of different chemicals called fatty acids and glycerol. Fat is used by living organisms as a good way of storing energy (calories) for later use.
Fibre	The indigestible constituent of plant foods, which form 'roughage' or bulk to the intestinal contents, and hence help to keep the intestinal peristalsis functioning and bowels opening normally.
Folic acid	An essential vitamin for the body's cells to work properly. Deficiency can particularly cause anaemia. Good food sources include liver and green vegetables.
Gastroenteritis	Usually due to an infection with a bacterium or virus from poorly cooked food or contaminated water. It results in vomiting and diarrhoea. Usually resolves without treatment. If a causative bacterium is cultured from the stool, specific antibiotics may be indicated.
Gastrointestinal tract	The long, flexible muscular tube which goes from the mouth to the anus. It includes the gullet, the stomach and the bowel (intestine). It allows food and drink to be digested and absorbed, and the waste to be passed out of the body.
Genes	Units of inheritance each made up of a string of chemicals (DNA) in the nucleus of each cell of our bodies, which vary from person to person.
Genetics	The study of how we inherit characteristics from one generation to the next, through our genes.
GFD (gluten-free diet)	A diet to treat people with coeliac disease. To be free of gluten, the food eaten must not contain wheat, barley, rye or their products.
Gliadin	The part of gluten which is soluble in an alcohol/water solution.
Gluten	The protein in the wheat seed which provides amino acids for the growing plant, or for a

human being when used as food. It provides much of the texture of flour when cooked.

Gluten challenge The deliberate ingestion of food containing a known amount of gluten in order to produce the symptoms or small intestinal mucosal abnormalities suggestive of coeliac disease. It is used when there is doubt about the definite diagnosis of coeliac disease.

Gluten-sensitive enteropathy An alternative name for coeliac disease, often used in North America.

Histology The study under the microscope of thin slivers of biological samples, including biopsies of human tissues.

Hordein The name for the gluten equivalent in barley.

Hyposplenism The state in which the spleen is not functioning properly. It is usually detected by finding some unusually shaped blood cells in the circulation, which are old and would normally have been removed by the spleen. Theoretically, a person with hyposplenism has a slightly increased risk of infections, but this is a very rare complication.

IgA/IgG/IgM Types of immunoglobulin.

Ileum The last part of the small intestine, which joins onto the large intestine (or colon).

Immune system The body's mechanism for protecting itself against 'foreign' substances. The action is sometimes misdirected against the body's own materials, and this is called auto-immunity.

Immunoglobulin A chemical produced by a type of lymphocyte called a plasma cell. There are three main types of immunoglobulin called A, G and M. They specifically bind to foreign substances, trying to eliminate them and are then called 'antibodies'.

Insulin *see* **Pancreas**.

Intraepithelial lymphocyte (IEL) A lymphocyte within the small intestinal epithelium, between enterocytes.

Irritable bowel syndrome (IBS)	A condition in which the bowel habit is erratic and associated with varying degrees of abdominal pain and often bloating, but without any recognizable other disease.
Jejunum	The mid-part of the small intestine, between the duodenum and the ileum.
Lactose	A type of sugar contained in milk and dairy products.
Lamina propria	The tissue of the mucosa which forms the core of the villi and surrounds the crypts.
Lymphocyte	A cell of the immune system which reacts against foreign substances in order to protect the body; there are several different types of lymphocyte.
Lymphoma	An uncontrolled multiplication of abnormal lymphocytes within the body, which are usually malignant (i.e. cancerous). Many are found to be circulating in the blood and collect in the lymph nodes, causing them to enlarge and be able to be felt.
Mucosa	The innermost layer of the intestine, consisting of fine blood vessels, fine nerves, immune cells and connecting tissue; covered by the epithelium.
Nucleus	The central, essential, particle of a living cell, which contains the genes.
Oesophagus (the gullet)	The first part of the gastrointestinal tract from the mouth to the stomach.
Osteomalacia	A bone disease due to deficiency of Vitamin D which results in bone with less calcium in it than normal. The bones are thus less rigid and can bend, and in children give the appearance seen in rickets.
Osteopenia	The earlier stage of osteoporosis when the reduced density of the bones is less severe.
Osteoporosis	A progressive disease of all the bones where they become less dense and weakened. There is a resulting increased risk of fracture.

Pancreas	An organ behind the stomach and close to the duodenum. It produces several chemicals, including insulin which passes into the blood to control the sugar levels. It also produces chemicals into the duodenum which begin the breakdown of food into simpler chemical substances.
Peptide	A short run of amino acids joined together.
Peristalsis	The normal forward movement of propulsion by the intestine, produced by its muscle layer.
Pneumococcal infection	An infection, usually pneumonia, caused by a particular bacterium (or bug) called streptococcus pneumoniae (or pneumococcus). It can usually be adequately treated with penicillin. However, severe infection can occur and can be dangerous, and other antibiotics may have to be used. Young children and elderly people are more prone to this infection.
Potential coeliac disease	A person with the genetic inheritance which predisposes them to develop coeliac disease on exposure to gluten, is said to have potential coeliac disease.
Prevalence	The frequency of something within a given number; for example, the number of cases of a disease within a specific number of the general population. The prevalence of coeliac disease is probably 1 in each 100 people in the general population.
Protein	A long run of amino acids joined together which forms a particular structure, for example, tissue fibres, walls of cells, enzymes (proteins which cause chemical reactions). Eating food which contains protein supplies the body with a source of nutrition and energy from the amino acids.
Refractory coeliac disease	A very rare form of coeliac disease. The small intestinal mucosa does not improve as expected with a gluten-free diet. Can occur in people

already diagnosed some time previously, who begin to deteriorate, or can be found in newly diagnosed patients. The patients can have severe gastrointestinal symptoms and poor nutrition.

Rye
A similar plant to wheat; its seeds are also grown to produce food.

Salt
A common mineral called sodium chloride (NaCl), naturally present in all living organisms and hence all food. It is an essential component of body fluids and is finely balanced by the body. Added to food, it acts as a preservative and enhances the taste, but too much can lead to ill health.

Screening
Testing a healthy population of people for the occurrence of a disease or abnormality.

Secalin
The name for the gluten equivalent in rye.

Sensitivity
The measure of how well a diagnostic test detects a disease when it is present. For example, 90 per cent sensitivity means the test detects the disease in 9 out of 10 cases, but misses 1 in 10; that is a 'false negative' result. The closer the sensitivity gets to 100 per cent the more sensitive (i.e. better) the test is.

Silent coeliac disease
Patients with the small intestinal abnormality typical of coeliac disease, but who have no, or very few, symptoms.

Small intestine
The long flexible muscular tube, about six metres long, which lies coiled up in the abdomen joining the stomach to the colon; its main function is to allow food to be digested and absorbed into the body.

Specificity
The measure of how often the result of a diagnostic test is negative when the disease is not present. For example, 90 per cent specificity means that in 9 out of 10 cases where the test is negative the patient does not have the

disease, but in 1 in 10 the test is positive when, in fact, the disease is not present; a 'false positive' result. The closer the specificity gets to 100 per cent the more specific (i.e. better) the test is.

Spleen
An organ in the left-hand side of the upper abdomen beneath the ribs. It is part of the immune system and helps to develop and store lymphocytes. It also removes and breaks down old cells in the circulating blood. People usually lead normal healthy lives if their spleen has to be removed for any reason.

Starch
The principal carbohydrate in food, especially in food from plants as opposed to animals.

Thyroid disorders
The thyroid gland in the neck produces the hormone thyroxine. Over-production causes excess activity of various bodily fonctions, leading to weight loss, hyperactivity, 'staring' eyes and anxiety. Under-production causes weight gain, slowing down, and feeling cold.

Tissue type
A way of distinguishing between humans by specific proteins on their cell surfaces. Some are more similar than others between different individuals, hence organ transplantation becomes possible.

tTG (tissue transglutaminase)
An enzyme in the body which is part of the endomysium tissue. An antibody almost identical to EMA is made against tTG but is easier to detect in a laboratory test. This is an anti-tTG antibody.

Ulcerative jejunitis
A very rare condition in which there are widespread ulcers in the small intestine. This leads to poor intestinal function with weight loss, malnutrition and severe diarrhoea. If it occurs, it is usually a rare complication of coeliac disease. Unfortunately, the outlook is poor.

Units of alcohol
These are defined as the equivalent amount of

pure alcohol (ethanol) in any particular volume of beverage. This obviously varies with the strength of the type of alcoholic drink. Thus one unit is present in a half pint of 'normal' strength beer or lager, or one 'moderate' size glass of wine, or one standard measure of spirits. It is easy to underestimate the amount of alcohol and therefore to drink more than imagined. The recommended safe limits per week are 21 units for men and 14 units for women.

Video capsule A very small device, the size of a medicine capsule. It contains a small camera and radio transmitter. After being swallowed it can take continuous pictures of the inside of the intestinal tract, which are recorded outside the body and can be viewed later. The capsule itself is used once, passed normally with food waste and flushed down the toilet.

Villus (plural villi) A finger-like projection of the small intestinal mucosa.

Vitamins An essential nutrient, required in small amounts, which the body itself cannot make and which therefore has to be obtained ordinarily from the diet.

Vitamin B$_{12}$ An essential vitamin for the body's cells to work properly. Deficiency can cause anaemia and nerve damage. Good sources include liver, meat and milk.

Vitamin D A vitamin required by humans to handle calcium and related substances in the body properly, hence its principal function is to maintain healthy bones. It is present in many foods and supplements, but is also made by the body in the skin when exposed to sunlight. Hence people who stay out of sunlight, cover up all their skin or have darker skin, make less of their own Vitamin D and are more likely to become deficient unless they have adequate dietary intake. Untreated coeliac patients are also more likely to become deficient because they do not absorb Vitamin D properly.

Wheat
A plant of the grass family. It is cultivated for its seeds which, when milled, constitute flour. A good source of nutrition, particularly carbohydrate, for humans.

Wheat starch
The principal constituent of flour, which is produced by milling wheat seeds.

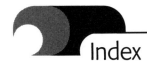

Index

Italic page numbers indicate figures not included in the text page range.

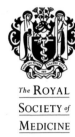

The Royal Society of Medicine (RSM) is an independent medical charity with a primary aim to provide continuing professional development for qualified medical and health-related professionals. The public benefits from health care professionals who have received high quality and relevant education from the RSM.

The Society celebrated its bicentenary in 2005. Each year it arranges and holds over 400 meetings for health care professionals across a wide range of medical subjects. In order to aid education and further training the Society also has the largest postgraduate medical library in Europe – based in central London together with online access to specialist databases. RSM Press, the Society's publishing arm, publishes books and journals principally aimed at the medical profession.

A number of conferences and events are held each year for the public as well as members of the Society. These include the successful 'Medicine and Me' series, designed to bring together patients, their carers and the medical profession. In addition, the RSM's Open and History of Medicine Sections arrange meetings on a regular basis which can be attended by the public.

In addition to the lectures and training provided by the RSM, members of the Society also have access to club facilities including accommodation and a restaurant. The conference and meeting facilities of the RSM were refurbished for their bicentenary and are available to the public for hire for meetings and seminars. In addition, Chandos House, a beautifully restored Georgian townhouse, designed by Robert Adam, is also now available to hire for training, receptions and weddings (as it has a civil wedding licence).

To find out more about the Royal Society of Medicine and the work it undertakes please visit www.rsm.ac.uk or call 020 7290 2991. For more information about RSM Press, please visit www.rsmpress.co.uk.